"In partnership with poets, places and practice, Francis Weller teaches us that it is time to know nothing, time to become immense, time to become seasoned adults through ritual and initiation, time to do our soul work, time to apprentice slowness and listen to trees, and time to, in the words of Rilke, let the future speak ruthlessly through us."

— ADRIENNE MAREE BROWN, author of *Emergent Strategy* and *Loving Corrections*

"As you [read this book], I suspect the world around you will begin to churn and curdle, and you might find yourself surrounded by a murmuring parliament of the rest of us welcoming you into the rough creases of our common descent."

—BAYO AKOMOLAFE, PhD, author of *These Wilds Beyond our Fences*

"The honesty that these essays ask of us is their greatest gift. What Francis Weller invites us to embrace in the Long Dark is not our valor and virtues so much as our colossal loss and grief."

—JOANNA MACY, author of *World As Lover, World As Self*

"Pierced by the multiple crises now roiling all earthbound lives, Francis Weller offers sober and elegant guidelines for facing the long dark rapids looming on our collective horizon. Come on down to the river. Pull up a log. Lean into the fire. Francis is here, casting spells and opening a hidden door to the animate underworld and to the unremembered sacred."

—BILL PLOTKIN, author of *Soulcraft* and *The Journey of Soul Initiation*

"With poetic and penetrating insight, Francis Weller invites us on a journey of the soul, one that reveals —in the dark passages of loss and grief— our collective immensity, belonging and luminosity."

—TARA BRACH, author of *Radical Acceptance* and *Radical Compassion*

"More than reading this book, . . . I want to live into the potential it envisions and share it with everyone I love. Weller bids us to embrace the journey into the realm of soul, dreams, mystery, imagination, and darkness, offering practical ways to weave the threads of medicine found there into our daily lives. In a muddled world, Weller brings clarity, wisdom, intimacy, reverence, and fluency with what the wild soul most wants. 'You are necessary,' he writes. 'It is time to become immense.'"

— ROSEMERRY WAHTOLA TROMMER, author of *The Unfolding* and host of *The Poetic Path*

IN THE
ABSENCE
OF THE
ORDINARY

Soul Work for
Times of Uncertainty

FRANCIS WELLER

North Atlantic Books
Huichin, unceded Ohlone land
Berkeley, California

North Atlantic Books
Huichin, unceded Ohlone land
2526 Martin Luther King Jr Way
Berkeley, California 94704 USA
www.northatlanticbooks.com

Cover art © Nosyrevy via Getty Images
Cover design by Jasmine Hromjak
Book design by Happenstance Type-O-Rama
List of Illustrations begin on page xi

Printed in Canada

In the Absence of the Ordinary: Soul Work for Times of Uncertainty is sponsored and published by North Atlantic Books, an educational nonprofit that collaborates with partners to develop cross-cultural perspectives; nurture holistic views of art, science, the humanities, and healing; and seed personal and global transformation by publishing work on the relationship of body, spirit, and nature.

North Atlantic Books's publications are distributed to the US trade and internationally by Penguin Random House Publishers Services. For further information, visit our website at *www.northatlanticbooks.com*.

The authorized representative in the EU for product safety and compliance is Eucomply OÜ, Pärnu mnt 139b-14, 11317 Tallinn, Estonia, hello@eucompliancepartner.com, +33757690241.

Library of Congress Cataloging-in-Publication Data

Names: Weller, Francis, 1956– author.
Title: In the absence of the ordinary : Soul Work for Times of Uncertainty / by Francis Weller.
Description: First. | Berkeley, CA : North Atlantic Books, [2025] | Includes bibliographical references and index.
Identifiers: LCCN 2024045614 (print) | LCCN 2024045615 (ebook) | ISBN 9798889842613 (trade paperback) | ISBN 9798889842620 (ebook)
Subjects: LCSH: Soul. | Rites and ceremonies. | Spiritual life.
Classification: LCC BL290 .W45 2025 (print) | LCC BL290 (ebook) | DDC 158.1—dc23/eng/20250213
LC record available at https://lccn.loc.gov/2024045614
LC ebook record available at https://lccn.loc.gov/2024045615

The interior of this book is printed on 100 percent recycled paper, and the cover includes material from well-managed forests.

2 3 4 5 6 7 8 9 FRIESENS 30 29 28 27 26 25

To the *Anima Mundi*,
the Soul of the World

The world and the gods are dead or alive according
to the condition of our souls.

—JAMES HILLMAN

CONTENTS

ILLUSTRATIONS

Introduction courtesy of powerofforever via Getty Images

Chapter One courtesy of ZU_09 via Getty Images

Chapter Two courtesy of Christine_Kohler via Getty Images

Chapter Three courtesy of benoitb via Getty Images

Chapter Four courtesy of clu via Getty Images

Chapter Five courtesy of bauhaus1000 via Getty Images

Chapter Six courtesy of NSA Digital Archive via Getty Images

Chapter Seven courtesy of ZU_09 via Getty Images

Chapter Eight courtesy of powerofforever via Getty Images

Chapter Nine courtesy of Thomas Faull via Getty Images

Chapter Ten courtesy of Christine_Kohler via Getty Images

Chapter Eleven courtesy of ilbusca via Getty Images

Chapter Twelve courtesy of powerofforever via Getty Images

Chapter Thirteen courtesy of powerofforever, via Getty Images

Chapter Fourteen courtesy of ilbusca via Getty Images

Chapter Fifteen courtesy of powerofforever via Getty Images

Chapter Sixteen courtesy of duncan1890 via Getty Images

Chapter Seventeen courtesy of ZU_09 via Getty Images

ACKNOWLEDGMENTS

ESSAYS ARE CURIOUS CREATURES, seemingly solitary, carrying a singular thread of intent and meaning. And yet, when gathered together, these essays revealed the hidden threads woven within each offering that combined to create a rich tapestry circulating around the ways of soul. This collection is rooted in the currents of sorrow, vulnerability, love, initiation, longing, and beauty. The imprints of soul are everywhere in these pages.

Many years ago, I had a dream where I am sitting at a kitchen table having a conversation with James Hillman. At one point, he gets up, walks over to a closet, and opens the door to reveal a chest of drawers. The drawers are very shallow, perhaps only an inch or two deep. He opens the drawers and takes out a piece of paper from each one. On the pages are the bibliographies of numerous authors, beginning with Carl Jung, folding back in time through Giambattista Vico and Marsilio Ficino, and on down to Heraclitus. He then turns to me and says, "This is your family tree." I have been claimed by this soul lineage. It is as much a part of me as my bloodline. It has fortified me for decades, offering a source of imagination and steady encouragement to follow the trail of soul. I stand on broad shoulders, full of gratitude for their enduring presence in my life.

I have been blessed with amazing mentors and teachers in my lifetime. I remember many afternoons sitting with Bob Griffin as he introduced me to a world of mystery and wonder. He was particularly adept at sending my mind down the rabbit hole with bewildering twists and turns, requiring me to let go of old stories and fictions. Clarke Berry is with me every day. He taught me the essential practices of patience and slowing down to the speed of soul. He was arguably the kindest man I ever knew. Bob Stein helped build the bridge between body and soul. His devotion to the holiness of our animal body is crucial to our collective healing. I am honored to have known these fine men. They, too, have gone on to become part of my soul lineage. Thank you all.

I have also been blessed with dear friends. Life has not been easy, and I often hid on the margins, hoping to slip by the gaze of the world. But there were a few who were able to find their way into my heart and who granted me shelter and a refuge within which I could risk being seen and known. Because of your love, my medicine found a way into the world. Richard Naegle, Doug von Koss, Larry Robinson, my soul brothers over the last thirty-five-plus years: I treasure our meetings. To my *Men of Spirit* brothers, Bob Hynes, John Meserve, Patrick Mullin: We have traveled many roads together. To the Blue Raven Village, my central place to go out from and come back to. I am also grateful to the Commonweal community, my other family, where I feel so welcome. And all of you who gathered with me to hold ritual space over the years: Katrina Mayo-Smith, Camie Velin, Kim Wylder, Kim Birdsong, Holly Truhlar, Alexandre Jodun, Erin Geesaman Rabke, Carl Rabke, Diane Dickinson, Judith Weller, and Kim Wardwell. Your presence there has been so valuable.

Thank you to Tim McKee and North Atlantic Books for the faith you showed in my writings. Our collaboration has been a rich source of encouragement. I am grateful for the skillful editing work done by Jasmine Respess. Your gentle touch kept faith with what was wanting to be said.

I carry an immense feeling of appreciation for the many people I have worked with over forty-two years in my psychotherapy practice and in countless communal ritual gatherings. I have learned from each of you how fully our lives are entangled with one another, with the stand of oaks, the night herons, the marginalized, the brokenhearted. I am especially grateful for all of you who have mentored with me, finding your unique ways of translating my work into new shapes and forms of service for our communities. Thank you and bless you for your fidelity to the work we are being called to do at this critical threshold time. As a mentor, this is a lasting gift to me.

Over the past decades, I have had the pleasure of working with many individuals devoted to the restoration of *living culture*. In particular, I have been moved by the commitment that our youth are showing in this time of uncertainty. Time and again, you have brought your grief, despair, longing, and conviction for our future to our ritual gatherings. I feel your passion and your commitment to work for a life that has meaning and beauty, belonging, and joy. I feel your longing to fashion a culture congruent with the ways and rhythms of the earth. I feel your creativity and wild imaginings, seeing things in ways my generation never dreamed of. You are powerful in the midst of your grief. You have been asked to carry so much, so soon, and the initiatory impulse may have been activated before you were ready. And maybe not. You may be the ones capable of finding a pathway through this collective dark night of the soul. All praise!

The thoughts and writings of many have influenced my work and understanding of these times: Carl Jung, James Hillman, Paul Shepard, Malidoma Somé, Thomas Berry, Gary Snyder, Terry Tempest Williams, Chellis Glendinning, Michael Meade, Joseph Campbell, Martín Prechtel, adrienne maree brown,

David Hinton, Thomas Moore, Linda Hogan, Joanna Macy, Derrick Jensen, Tara Brach, bell hooks, Robert Bly, Kathleen Dean Moore, David Abram, and all the others who have shown me the ways to live a life of meaning.

Deep gratitude to all the ancestors, human and more-than-human. The immense inheritance that resides within your halls is a source of inspiration and guidance during these times of uncertainty. Calling upon this residual wisdom grants us a sense of direction and faith that we can find our way through the Long Dark.

I want to acknowledge all my kin, rooted in blood and soul, dream and soil. This landscape is saturated with beauty and sorrow, awe and suffering. It shimmers with the sacred and is a constant reminder of our wider intimacies that we are invited to foster and nourish. Our spiritual responsibility is to remember our kinship ties and to offer gratitude for the ongoing blessings that arise from the living cosmos.

And lastly, a profound thank you to my wife, Judith. You have participated in the many iterations of these essays, adding your reflections, thoughts, outrage, humor, and love to every one of them. This is a co-creation nourished by your intuitive wisdom and imagination. They are an offering from our *third body*.

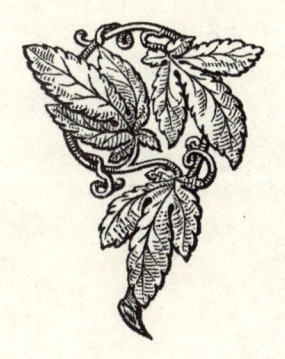

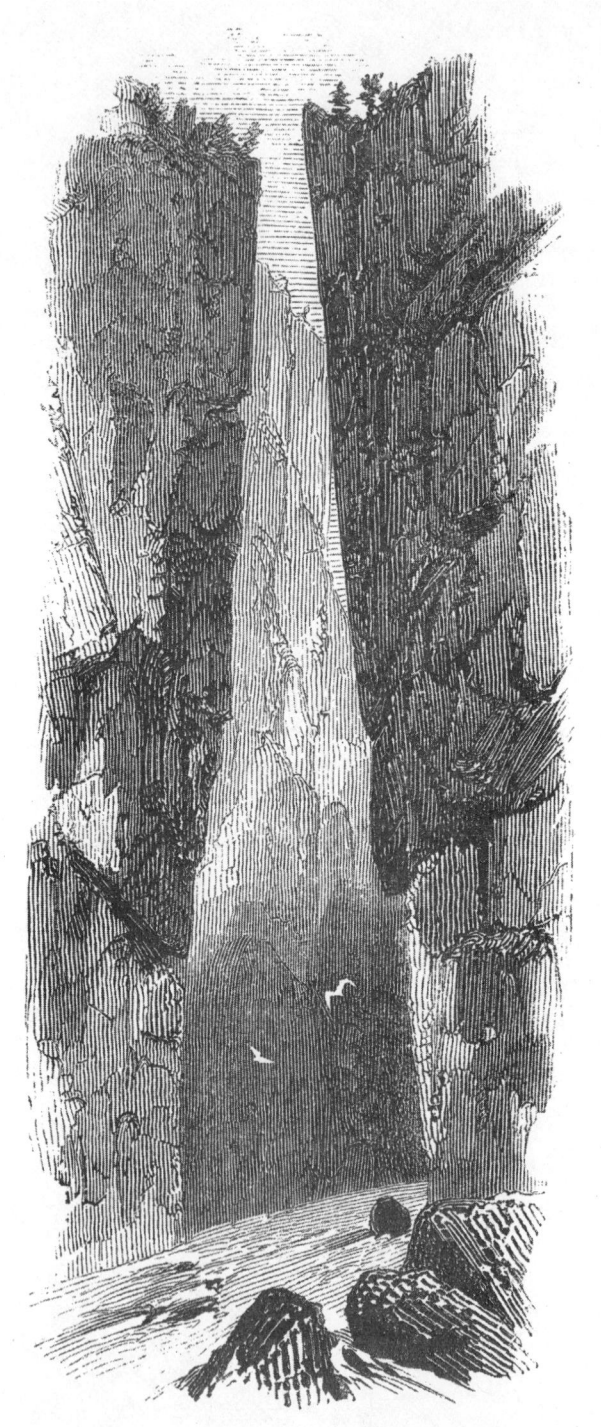

INTRODUCTION
In the Absence of the Ordinary

DAY BY DAY, we shape a life. Sometimes rather aimlessly, and at other times with deliberation and intention. The more we pay attention, the more we notice the many ordinary moments that add texture and meaning to our lives. Greeting a friend on the street; a shared meal; a quiet walk in the woods; going to the market or gazing at the night sky. Nothing special. Simply the ordinary rounds of coming and going, connection and engagement. We depend upon these gestures to sustain the currency of belonging.

These days, however, the felt sense of continuity and participation in our day-to-day world has been radically altered. When the pandemic emerged in 2020, the experience of the familiar was eclipsed as much of the world came to an abrupt stop. In addition, the growing impact of climate disruption, cultural fragmentation, regional conflicts, and economic uncertainty has crashed into our psychic lives adding to the feeling that we are not living in ordinary times. We can no longer divide the world *out there* from the world *in here*. It is becoming increasingly clear that our lives are completely entangled with the living fabric of the world. How could they not be?

In truth, we have entered a prolonged season of *descent* that has taken us down into a different geography. It is a time of gravity and extremes as we witness the hottest temperatures on record, inflamed political discourse, the fraying of social bonds, and the emerging reality of widespread species extinction. In the imagery of myth and fairy tales, we have left the ordinary world and have entered the *underworld*, a sightless terrain that is shadowy and strange. The underworld is a place of dream and imagination, of gestation and mystery, of uncertainty and silence. This move into the underworld has left our sense of bearing dislodged. We don't fully know where we are at this moment in our shared story. We must learn to get quiet and still. We must develop our capacity to see with what Zen teacher and author Susan Murphy calls the "dark adapted eye."[1]

In this shadowed terrain, we encounter a landscape familiar to soul—loss, grief, death, uncertainty, vulnerability, and fear. We have—in the old language of alchemy—crossed into the *nigredo*, the blackening. The alchemists described this time as a season of decay, of shedding and endings, of falling apart and undoing. It is not difficult to see these are the conditions of our world. This is not a time of rising and growth. It is not a time of confidence and ease. No. We are hunkered down. "Down" being the operative word. *From the perspective of soul, down is holy ground.*

Collectively, we are not familiar with descent as something valued and essential and most assuredly not something we consider holy. Most of us live in an ascension culture. We love things rising up . . . up . . . up . . . always up. We value success and strength, power and prowess. When things begin to go down, we can feel panic, uncertainty, and even dread. How can we meet these unpredictable times with a sense of courage and faith? Courage to keep our hearts open to face the world as it is and faith that something meaningful lingers in the descent. How can we, once again, come to see the holiness that dwells in the darkness?

To remember the sacredness in the dark, it is important that we become fluent in the manners and ways of soul. By soul I am referring more to a way of seeing than to some metaphysical reality. I hold soul from an archetypal perspective, following in the long lineage that flows through James Hillman and Carl Jung, down through the poetic traditions, an animist sensibility, and into indigenous mind. Soul draws us downward, into the geography of vulnerability, tenderness, loss, intimacy, and death. It keeps us close to longing, beauty, ritual, outrage, and the forest of the imagination. Soul circulates through the terrain of wounds and suffering, close to the broken heart, keeping us near to what is found on the margins, both internally and culturally. Soul is both deeply interior, offering us a sense of who we are most authentically, and simultaneously communal at the same time. Soul navigates the twining trail between sovereignty and intimacy. To know soul is to feel our wild entanglement with all things, revealing our ongoing relationship with the *anima mundi*, the soul of the world.

As we descend ever farther into the collective unknown, into the underworld, we are called to remember the *disciplines of soul* that may enable us to navigate through what I have come to call the *Long Dark*. Primary among these disciplines is the practice of *deep listening*, which acknowledges the wisdom in others and in the dreaming Earth. When we listen deeply, we begin to uncover what wants to be brought into awareness. We become receptive and permeable to sources of wisdom that lie beyond the purely human. Listening is the art of reverence. The Inuit living north of the Arctic Circle have a word in their language, *qarrtsiluni*, which translates "Sitting together in the darkness, waiting for something to happen or burst forth." This expectant attitude is rich with deep listening, aching to hear the song that will provide for the village.

A second discipline that is essential for these times is *restraint*.*
Restraint offers a breath, a pause, a moment of reflection, which
allows things to be revealed. Restraint enables something to ripen
before we move into action. Additionally, *humility* honors our
mutuality and brings us close to the ground, a gesture that keeps
us aware of our entanglement with the living world.

A further discipline we need to develop is our capacity to
embrace *not knowing*. Not knowing reminds us that we live in
mystery, an ever-unfolding, unshaped moment. When we drop
into the space of not knowing, we are able to suspend our con-
trived expectations we so readily rely upon. We become suscep-
tible to mystery, to revelation. We do not know what is going to
happen, and this truth keeps us humble, vulnerable, and open
to possibilities. Not knowing situates us at the edge of discovery, especially when we are in the uncharted waters of the underworld. And finally . . . *letting go* . . . rooted in the fundamental
truth of impermanence. Each of us is preparing for our own disappearance as well as witnessing the constantly shifting world.
We are reminded of the continual process of change. Letting go
of control, outcomes, and certainty softens the space between us
and all the others with whom we share this shimmering world.

Each of these disciplines helps us to cultivate our presence in
the underworld of the Long Dark.

I have spent the last four decades tracking the movements of
soul, most especially through the lairs of grief. In my practice as
a psychotherapist and in many workshops, I have seen the wide
range of sorrows that we carry in our hearts. From early traumas,

---

* See chapter 9, "The Gift of Restraint."

deaths, divorces, suicides of beloved family or friends, addictions, illnesses, and more . . . the "size of the cloth" has become painfully apparent. More and more frequently, I hear in the laments of individuals, not so much grief for their personal losses but for the wider, wilder world that is being diminished minute by minute. They are registering in their souls the sorrows of the world. Strangely, this gives me hope.

We have clearly entered the Long Dark. It may be decades or more likely a few generations before we see the farther shore of this crisis, if we make it. I say this not with a note of despair, or with an attitude of hopelessness, but, instead, recognizing and valuing the necessary work that takes place in the dark. It is the realm of soul—of whispers and dreams, mystery and imagination, death and ancestors. It is an essential territory, both inevitable and required, offering a form of soul gestation that may gradually give shape to our deeper lives, personally and communally. Certain things can happen only in this grotto of darkness. Think of the wild network of roots and microbes, mycelia, and minerals, making possible all that we see in the day world, or the extensive networks within our own bodies, bringing blood, nutrients, oxygen, and thought to our corporeal lives. All of it happening in the darkness.

We must become fluent in the manners and ways of soul. In addition to the disciplines of soul, we are required to develop a potent set of skills as we descend ever farther into the collective unknown. We are being asked to hone the faculties of soul that will enable us to navigate through the Long Dark. Skills such as ritual literacy, initiation practices to support our youth in their movements toward adulthood, the shaping of elders, maintaining relations with the invisible world of ancestors and the sacred, all contribute to a vital and robust ground of living culture.

Primary among the skills we will need to cultivate is our capacity to grieve. My previous writings have focused on the way grief and loss touch our personal lives. From the deaths of loved ones to the loss of homes or relationships to the shattering experience of trauma, we are visited by sorrow in many ways. In these current times, we have entered a new constellation in which our grief is often collective. *Grief will be the keynote for the foreseeable future.* We are in a deep dive into the unknown, riddled with pockets of loss. Homes, health, security, community, and even our basic trust in the future are now in question. COVID-19 forced this into our consciousness, but this truth has been there for some time now, embedded in the emerging climate crisis and the eroding of the social fabric of culture. We have been quickened by the cumulative changes to realize a vital truth: We are in a *rough initiation*.

Fear and anxiety readily appear in times like these when the ground of the ordinary is unsettled. Our work is to turn toward these jittery guests and make a place at the table to offer tea and soup, a warm place to rest. Grief will also come knocking as our plans and expectations of normalcy fade into shadows, and we are left with our faith in the world being shaken. This is a loss worthy of our attention and kindness. Our times remind us of something inevitable but strangely denied: we are vulnerable, interdependent animals, clinging delicately to our little thread of life. The old Zen phrase "Not knowing is most intimate" rings true. We do not know what will happen today or tomorrow, and this brings us to the intimate truth of our mutual tender existence.

We are tumbling through a rough initiation. Radical alterations are occurring in our inner and outer landscapes. It is simultaneously deeply personal and wildly collective, binding us to one another. Everyone we meet in the grocery store, in line at the gas station, walking their dog, is tangled up in this liminal space betwixt and between the familiar world and the strange, emergent one. Hang on!

Much is asked of us during threshold times like these. In my work with the Commonweal Cancer Help Program, I often hear how lost someone feels once they receive the diagnosis, undergo treatment, and become a part of the medical machinery that often consumes much of their daily routine. The frequent lament is "I don't know who I am anymore." This is the deep work of initiation. It is meant to dislodge our old identity, the sediment of self that we affix to our sense of who we are. We are meant to be radically changed by these encounters. We do not want to come out of these turbulent times the same as we went in. That is the invitation in this moment of history: radical change that nourishes the life force of the commons.

So now what? How do we navigate this tidal surge of uncertainty? How do we engage the world in the absence of the ordinary? Our first move could be to reimagine our times as necessary. I like to imagine that the immune response of the world is being activated by the various threats and harm stirring in the field. And what if you and I are cells within the immune system, adding our voice, our actions, our affection to the situation. What if this is true? What if this matters?

What else? Can we coax a few words of praise from our lips? Perhaps recite a poem to the birds, plant seeds, call a friend, pray, read the great myths that tell us, again and again, how we might find our way through the impossible. This is a season of remembering the ancient rhythms of soul. It is a time to become immense.

To become immense means to recall how embedded we are in an animate world—a world that dreams and enchants, a world that excites our imaginations and conjures our affections through its stunning beauty. Everything we need is here. We only need to remember the wider embrace of our belonging to woodlands and prairies, marshlands, and neighborhoods, to the old stories and the tender gestures of a friend. To become immense also includes the radical act of welcoming all of who we are into the story. Nothing excluded. We become large through accepting all aspects of our being—weakness and need, loneliness and sorrow, shame and fear—everything seen as essential to our wholeness, our immensity.

Fear can rattle us and activate strategic patterns of survival when the ground of the ordinary crumbles. These patterns enabled us to endure in our lifetimes, but they cannot help us across this tremulous initiatory threshold we face as a wider community. For that, we need to amplify the potency of the adult. As is true of any genuine initiation, it requires the ripening of our being and stepping more fully into our robust identity rooted in soul. We become immense, not in some grandiose, "I've got this" kind of way, but in a way where we become flexible like a willow, taking it all into our open arms and offering shelter to all that is frightened and vulnerable.

James Hillman, the brilliant archetypal psychologist, wrote, "The world and the gods are dead or alive according to the condition of our souls."[2] In other words, the vitality of the animate, sensuous world and our encounter with the sacred depend on our souls being fully alive! A soul that is awake is entangled with the living world—its beauty, allure, and wonder, its sorrows, rips, and tears. The condition of our soul matters!

So, let us return to simple things: stillness, story, beauty, compassion, and patience. This will not resolve quickly. The Long Dark will be with us for some time. Ritual, prayer, meditation, and creativity are ways to foster an intimacy with the world of soul and the soul of the world.

Many of the great myths began in a time such as this. The land has become barren; the king, corrupted; the ways of peace, lost. It is in these conditions that a ripeness arises in the soul for deep-rooted change. Soul responds to crisis by awakening to a deeper sense of purpose, leaning into how it can contribute to the repair and renewal of the world.

When the ordinary fades, when the familiar rhythms and patterns of shared living erode, something is activated within the soul. Hidden invitations and initiations arise in a time of uncertainty. The soul recognizes the markers of descent—darkness, sorrow, anxiety—as requiring radical change. The conditions of trouble and uncertainty activate some profound movement toward alterations in the psychic landscape. These are the precise times when the possibility for shifts in the collective field occurs. We are in such a threshold time. We are being called to embody courage and humility. Every one of us will be affected by the changes wrought by this difficult visitation. Carl Jung said that each of us is a makeweight in the affairs of the world. Never think that you have nothing to contribute to the shaping of our future. You are needed. You are necessary. It is time to become immense.

The essays and reflections in this collection were written over the years, often in response to local or cultural experiences, like the pandemic and the wildfires that erupted in California and across the planet. I originally gathered them together to offer some solace during the highly uncertain times that accompanied the arrival of COVID. That uncertainty has not diminished over the years. The threads of soul that are held and woven together in these essays offer a sense of how we may respond to the deep unknown that is unfolding around us. The vital strands of initiation, the Long Dark, grief work, ritual, practice, community, and beauty help us to hold these times with a soulful bearing. These essays are a response, a prayer, an offering to the times we are in. They form a primer on ways to hold this time through practices rooted in soul. May they offer you some ground upon which to find rest in these unsettled times. Stay safe. Stay well. Stay connected.

FRANCIS WELLER

Russian River Watershed

PART I

&

When the Bough Breaks

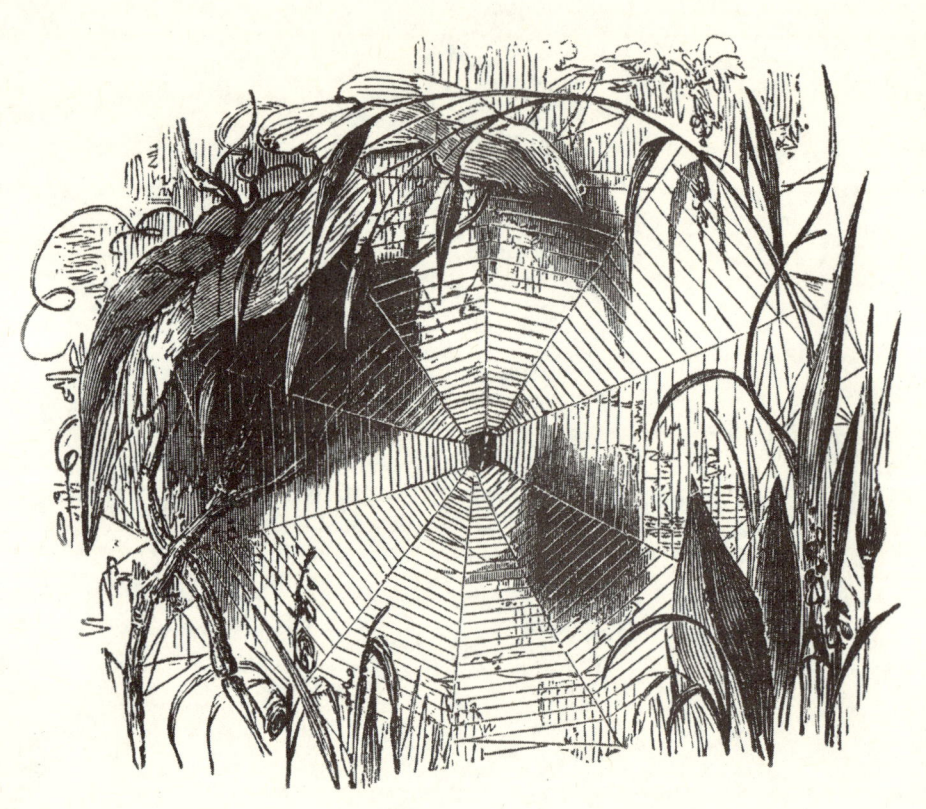

One

Rough Initiations

SEVERAL YEARS AGO, I wrote an article called "The Movements That Made Us Human," in which I related an experience I had learning to flint knap: the making of arrowheads and spearpoints from stone. In the process of learning this ancient skill, a body memory flickered into my awareness: we have been making this gesture, this exact movement of lifting stone above our heads and striking down on stone, for more than one million years. This movement, along with others, such as making fire, making cordage, tracking game, basket making, communal rituals, initiation, and storytelling, are what slowly gave shape to our psychic and communal lives. We have made these movements generation upon generation and now, in the barest wisp of a moment, we have stopped. What happens to our psyches, to our very beings, in the absence of these movements? What happens to our cultures when these sturdy and reliable rhythms go silent?

Entire areas of our nature remain inactivated. By extension, entire areas of the commons of right relations and good manners with the living world are also missing. These movements were highly engaged with the surrounding world: gathering plants for baskets and cordage; tracking deer, bison, and antelope; tending the passages from youth into adulthood through sacred initiations; all were done with an attitude of reverence. By silencing these movements, a distinct language of intimacy with the enveloping world has been lost. This strikes a profound note in the collective hum of grief.

One of the essential movements that made us human was our ability to hold one another in times of grief and trauma. This skill has, for the most part, been lost under the extreme weight of individualism and privatization. This has had a profound impact on how we process and metabolize our personal encounters with loss and intense emotional experiences. Without the familiar and reliable container of community and family, these times can penetrate our psychic lives in a shattering way, leaving us shaken, frightened, and unsure of our next footstep. This is the experience of trauma. Trauma is any encounter, acute or prolonged, that overwhelms the capacity of the psyche to process the experience. In these times, what confronts us is too intense to hold, integrate, or comprehend. The emotional charge that arises saturates our capacity to make sense of the experience, and we become overwhelmed and often feel utterly alone.

We have become familiar with the term PTSD (post-traumatic stress disorder). We hear stories of veterans returning from war carrying the violence they experienced and witnessed within them. Natural disasters, car accidents, school shootings, rape, or the sudden death of someone we love can all cause acute trauma. The psychic load of these experiences lodges deep within victims' bodies.

There are other forms of trauma as well. Trauma can also arise in our psyches, not so much from an event but through erosion; the slow wearing away of the sense of trust, security, and worth through prolonged exposure to neglect, abandonment, or shaming. This is what is called *developmental trauma* or what I call *slow trauma*.

What makes an experience traumatic, in addition to the pain of the encounter, is the absence of an adequate holding environment capable of supporting us in these times. Pain itself is not pathological. The pathology emerges from the isolation that all too often surrounds our experience. What we needed in these times were attuned and attentive individuals who could sense the distress we were experiencing and offer us assurance, soothing, and safe touch to help us re-modulate our inner states. A holding environment is a form of ritual ground, within which we can pour our grief, fear, and pain and trust that it will be held.

Trauma is inherent in being human. From suffering and loss to broken hearts and betrayals, we will all encounter many moments of trauma. In the absence of the village—which was the original holding environment—these times settle like sediment in our beings, taking on a feeling of overwhelm and frequently of shame. It is as if we intuitively know that someone should have responded to our distress, and when they did not show up, the thought fell on us like ash that it must be because of our unworthiness. It confirms our lack of welcome and belonging, reinforcing our isolation and exile.

In my work as a psychotherapist, I have seen many people who were experiencing circumstances that profoundly affected their lives—life-threatening illnesses, the lingering effects of neglect in childhood, violations to body and soul through rape or molestation, or the haunting remains of war. In their stories, I began to see the parallels between their traumatic experience and traditional initiation. I began to call their experiences "rough initiations" to provide a greater context for what happened to them. Seeing these encounters as the ordeal that *activated an initiatory process* granted them a way to hold what was occurring in their lives with compassion and warmth: an essential shift in the way the material was being held.

In any genuine initiatory experience and in all truly traumatic events, the following circumstances occur:

- We leave the world that was known. The diagnosis, the accident, the death of a beloved, all shatter the world we once occupied.

- There is a radical alteration in our sense of self. The familiar self is shaken and disrupted. We don't know who we are anymore.

- There is a realization that nothing will ever be the same. We can never return to the world that was. We are left radically changed by the encounter.

Traditional initiation occurred outside the familiar landscape of family and friends, the daily rounds of meals, and work. It occurred in a time outside time. What was known and accustomed was left behind as the initiate entered a strange and unpredictable world while simultaneously being held within the sacred container of community. For the cancer patient, the soldier, the victim of rape, or the child of neglect, the world takes on new hues, colored by the wash of pain and terror that accompanies their experience. They too have entered an alternate reality, yet one devoid of the sacred container of ritual and village. In this unfamiliar and often frightening terrain, they encounter the unraveling of their known existence.

Ritual initiation radically reshapes our sense of self. It is meant to break us open to the widest possible experience in identity. This shift in identity shows itself in times of trauma as well. I hear the phrase "I don't know who I am anymore" every time I meet with the participants in the Cancer Help Program. The same is true for other forms of trauma as well, shaking individuals to the core, and reducing the arc of identity.

In an ideal situation, identity slowly emerges from the rich loom of inner and outer threads, woven together to craft something unique and beautiful. Until the age of initiation, the coalescing self is meant to be sheltered, protected, and allowed to burrow deep into the womb of family and village. This identity, however, is not large enough to contain the wild edge of the soul's calling or the demands of the daimon. *When the safety of the familiar confronts the yearnings of the soul, it is time for initiation.* It is a time of disruption and eruption as the demands of the soul make themselves known. It is at this point that the elders recognized the need to end the life of the youth, as they knew it, and ritually escort them across the threshold into a new sense of self.

Trauma enacts the same shifts in identity, often without the guidance, witnessing, and containment of the village. This free-fall experience can leave us feeling as though we have little sense of who we are any longer. And now, no matter how hard we try, we cannot put the pieces together again. We cannot go back to how things were before the cancer diagnosis, the accident, the war, the hurricane, or the death of our child: Nothing will ever be the same; and too often, we are asked to carry it alone, in silence.

Traditional initiation is what I call a *contained encounter with death*. Initiates were often put through a series of intense ordeals such as prolonged fasting, being buried overnight, or dancing for hours until the body collapsed from exhaustion. Death is ever-present during initiation, signaling to the initiate the gravity of the moment. These ordeals dislodge the current sense of self and radically reshape it through encounters with vastly larger energies. No amount of personal strength or control can outlast the conditions that are evoked by the ritual process of initiation. Only by releasing the old forms will something emerge on the other side. The initiate, in a very real sense, dies and is rebirthed at the end of this process into a wider cosmological story and identity. They have died to the solely personal and have entered the sacred dimension of mythic life.

Traditionally, initiation was never meant for the individual. It had nothing to do with personal growth or self-improvement. It was an act of sacrifice on behalf of the greater community into which the initiate was brought and to which they now hold allegiance. They were being made ready to step into their place of maintaining the vitality and well-being of the village, the clan, the watershed, the ancestors, and spirit. It was never about them, but about the continuum of generations to come.

This thought is exceedingly difficult for us to digest in our highly personalized/psychologizing way of thinking and perceiving. It is always about us—our wounds, our growth—which keeps us at the center of the wheel. Traditional initiation, in contrast, breaks us into a wider and more inclusive experience of self. We become part canyon, part meadowlark, part cloud bank, part village. We are made porous through these profoundly deranging experiences, broken open to allow ourselves to be penetrated by the holiness that pervades all things. Through this communion, we feel our kinship with the singing, breathing world/cosmos. We become immense and connected to the whole. We fall in love with the world and learn to protect what we love.

I called initiation "a contained encounter with death." Martín Prechtel said those "who didn't fight death in adolescence were destined to live in a walking death."[3] This failure to confront death during initiation dooms many of us to become agents of death, eating life wherever we go. Any sideways glance at our culture reveals a massively consumptive, parasitic energy, feeding off the life force of the planet. This is the direct consequence of abandoning the essential practice of initiation.

Restoring rituals of initiation is at the heart of any meaningful cultural change.

Trauma, in contrast, is an *uncontained encounter with death*. Few, if any, of the conditions needed to meaningfully process the trauma were present. We felt naked and exposed to the bitter winds of neglect or violence. Our internal environment shifted and rearranged itself in our attempts to mediate these extreme states. We withdrew from the world, found ways to ease our distress, and sought security from anyone we could convince to grant us provisional shelter. We established sentinels at the periphery of awareness to keep us safe and always kept a vigilant watch. We were reshaped by these traumatic times. It became difficult to regulate our inner worlds, which could be suddenly tossed about by any event in our life.

I know in my own life, the neglect and violence I experienced made me wary and distrusting of love, certain that it was fleeting at best and certain to disappoint. I leaned heavily on distraction and dissociation to remain at a safe distance from my pain and grief. Eventually, however, the soul finds cracks in the foundation and brings to the surface what we attempted to bury, in hopes of completing the initiation that remained latent in the trauma. *Our wounds carry within them the unripened seeds of initiation.*

The German word for trauma is *seelenershuetterung*, which means "soul-shaking." This feels more alive than the clinical word "trauma." We are shaken in times of trauma, disoriented, and bewildered. Edward Tick, author of *War and the Soul*, wrote that "The Hopi people call trauma *tsawana*, meaning 'a state of mind that is in terror,'" and "The Lakota called trauma *nagi napayape*, meaning, 'the spirits leave him.'"[4] Trauma enters our beings at profoundly deep levels, not unlike the conditions of initiation. However, without the mediating conditions that contained traditional initiation processes, these experiences leave us shattered and alone—the exact opposite end of the spectrum that accompanies initiation. Whereas initiation breaks us open to the widest possible aperture of inclusion in connection to the breathing cosmos, trauma isolates us and fragments us into the smallest imaginable hub of existence. One man shared that his goal was to live at or below zero; to take up no room in the world since he had no right to be here.

Trauma leaves us thinned and exhausted. Strategies of survival consume much of our life energy. The condition that befalls us following trauma resembles, in a powerful way, what traditional cultures call *soul loss*. This was the most feared condition for Indigenous people. It led to a flattened world, disenchanted, and emptied of vitality, joy, and passion. Relations with the living, singing world become muted in this condition, leaving one stranded in a deadened world.

Soul loss is experienced as a depletion of our vital essence, leading to a decreased sense of potency and power. In mythological imagery, we have entered the *wasteland*. Here, images appear in dreams of ghettos and prisons, ragged orphans, and barren stretches of empty buildings. Psychologically we call this depression, but to the indigenous soul, depression is the symptom, not the illness. The illness is soul loss and that is not amenable to medication.

To heal from our traumas, from soul loss, we must restore the conditions that offer something alluring and compelling to coax the soul back home. In other words, what reconstitutes the psyche after trauma, in addition to understanding what happened, is reestablishing our place within the wider cosmological context. We must be restored and re-storied to complete the rough initiation that was precipitated by the trauma. In other words, we must return to our lives as vital and engaged participants in the deep song of the world.

For many years, I had the honor of leading the *Men of Spirit* initiation process, a yearlong intensive rite of passage. What I began to understand from the work we were doing, and from studying initiations in other cultures, is that a certain set of variables must be in place to contain the encounter with death and make the transition possible from youth to adult. *These same conditions are what help us restore the psyche after trauma.*

1. **It requires a certain context: Community.** Initiation is meaningless outside of the village. We need something to serve: We do this for the sake thereof. In other words, initiation was not meant for the sake of the individual; it was done for the welfare of the greater circle to which they belong. Initiates returned to the village, the community or tribe, as newly created members of the wider cosmos. They were now authorized to participate in the care and maintenance of the community.

    Similarly, a traumatized individual needs to feel the arms of the community holding them in their extreme condition. Through the eyes and hearts of the circle, the violated soul can begin to feel the resonance that is available to them inviting them home.

2. **It requires a certain energetic: Ritual.** Ritual is a highly focused process that provides sufficient heat to cook the soul. The particular gestures, which are unique to each culture, are guided by ritual elders. Ritual invites the potential for derangement—the process of shaking us out of the agreed-upon constructs of family/culture and into a larger, soul-based sense of living. The community requires potent adults who are guardians of their own sovereignty.

    Traditionally, ritual was the means by which the community helped to restore a person or the community to wellness following any traumatic event. It was the original regulating process for healing.

3. **It requires a certain vibration: The Sacred.** Ritual opens us to the Mystery, the invisible world of the sacred. Initiation without the engagement of the sacred fails to open us to our expanded sense of identity. It requires invisible allies and energies to help us slip off the coat of our small lives. Through this encounter, we begin a lifelong courtship of the holy.

   Acknowledging the presence of the sacred extends the bonds of connectivity into the unseen dimensions of life. This is a vital move that reminds us we are a part of the living cosmos.

4. **It requires a certain spaciousness: Time.** Many initiatory processes last six weeks to six months out in the bush. During this prolonged time, all ties to the familiar are broken and you enter the cocoon of your own disappearance. This takes time. This alternative rhythm enables the psyche to let go of the conditioned cadence that accompanies daily life. We need to slip into soul time, "geologic time," as my mentor Clarke Berry called it. This expanded sense of time allowed the timeless to break through, offering glimpses of the eternal that rooted the new life of the initiate in something vast.

5. **It requires a certain terrain: Place.** Initiation occurs in place, a geography with familiar hills, caves, trees, and rivers. Traditionally, mythic places, where the old ones gave shape to the landscape, were the grounds upon which the initiates were taken, providing an ancestral root to their own experiences. Now watersheds, a bioregion particular to our being, are the terrain into which we are invited. We

are initiated into place as surely as we are into our communities. Place is very particular. We can see this today when Indigenous people are fighting to the death to protect their lands from oil and mining companies. To these traditional people, self and land are one.

When these five elements are woven together, the container is fortified, and we are able to cross the threshold and enter into our own adult lives with the capacity of honoring life and feeding the soul of the world. These primary constituents help to stabilize the internal processes of self-attunement, self-regulation, and our capacity to more readily hold steady in our adult life. We begin to suture the tears in our coat of belonging.

For example, a study of Native American and non-Native American soldiers returning from the Afghanistan and Iraq wars was revealing. It showed that the soldiers who participated only in conventional PTSD treatments had a 40 percent success rate for the treatment. However, those soldiers who participated in traditional Native practices, such as sweat lodges, pipe ceremonies, and vision quests, had a 72 percent success rate in recovering from their symptoms.[5] The difference was the restoration of the cosmological ground—the soldiers returned to the larger field of belonging. In the Indigenous understanding, it is impossible to separate body, mind, soul, and spirit. Any approach to healing must include all these aspects of our being. What is worth noting is that when non-Native soldiers were offered the same rituals, they also experienced an increase in recovery from the trauma.

The most neglected aspect in our encounters with initiatory experiences is the lack of an adequate return. Severance without the possibility of return is permanent exile. Healing trauma requires a restoration of the matrix of life. Trauma often lingers in our bodies and souls as a *suspended initiation*. What began when the rupture occurred must now be rejoined and completed.

When we return to the wounds, we reignite the suspended initiatory process and help to complete the crossing into a new state of being. This is not easy or quick. It depends upon a slow, deliberate titration of energy from the liminal world, the betwixt and between state, that signals to the psyche that we have found our way through the maelstrom of radical change. This is the process of homecoming. When we are able to return to the original ground of our belonging, we come home and remember who we are, where we belong, and what is sacred.

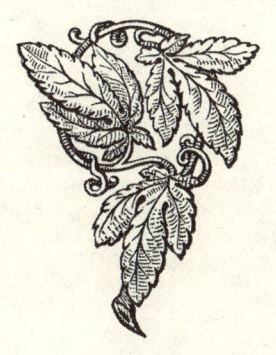

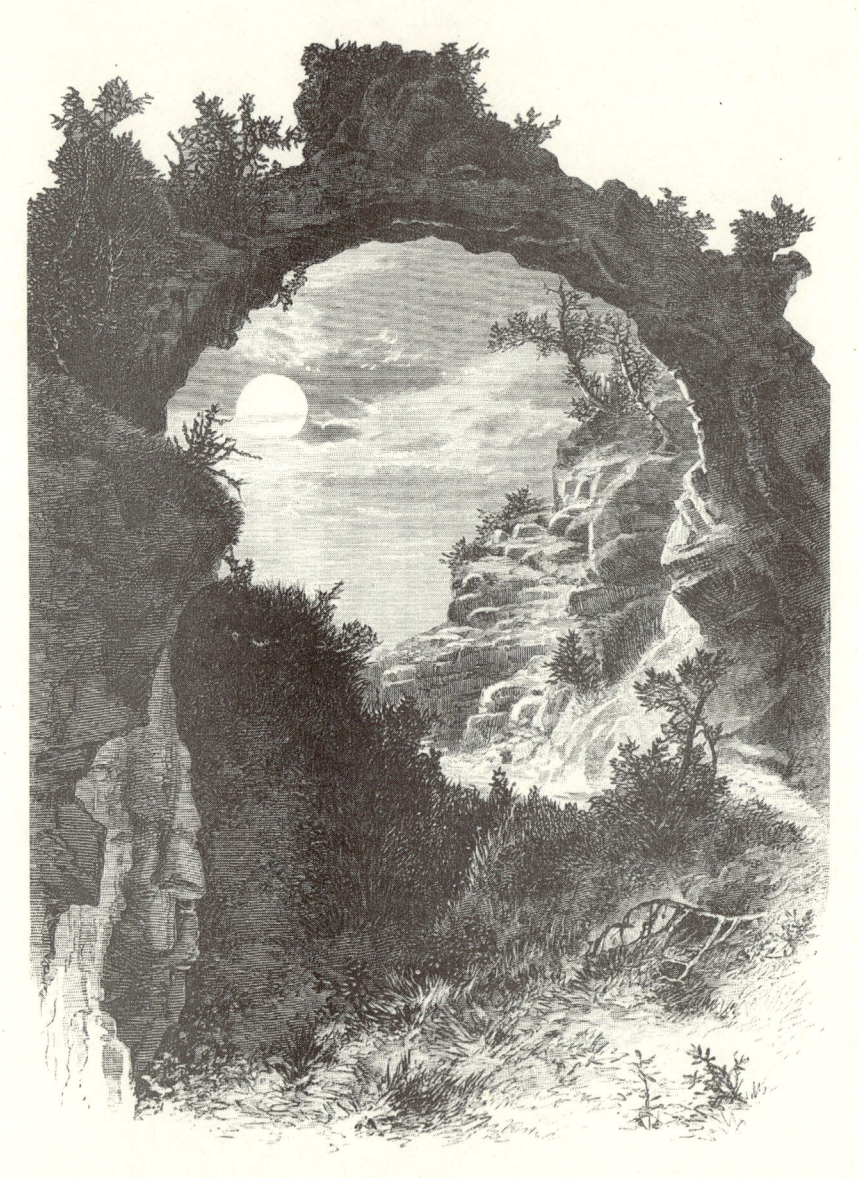

Two

Some People Wake Up
Reflections on Initiation

Again and again
Some people wake up.
They have no ground in the crowd
And they emerge according to broader laws.
They carry strange customs with them,
And demand room for bold gestures.

The future speaks ruthlessly through them.[6]
—RAINER MARIA RILKE

NO DOUBT YOU have noticed that we are living in turbulent times culturally and as a planet. All pretense of immunity is collapsing as we realize how completely entangled our lives are with one another, with kelp beds and calving glaciers, with refugees and the dreams of young people everywhere. The disequilibrium shaking the world feels like a continual tremor on the fault lines of our psychic lives. Very few things feel stable. It is like a fever dream. It may be that this is the initiatory threshold we require to wake us up. Whatever is happening, much will be asked of us if we are to make it through the whitewater of this narrow passage. We do not know what lies ahead, but one thing is sure: This is a time for bold gestures. It is time to wake up and humbly take our place on this stunning planet. The future is speaking ruthlessly through us.

The immediate need of our time is for ripened and seasoned adult human beings to take their place in our communities; individuals who carry a deep and abiding fidelity to the living body of this benevolent earth, to beauty, and to their own souls. Traditionally, these were the ones who had successfully crossed a series of initiatory thresholds and had come through as protectors and carriers of the communal soul. They were the ones whose artistry and wisdom kept the current of culture alive. We live in a society that has all but abandoned rituals of initiation. Consequently, we are languishing from the absence of mature and robust adults.

How do we become seasoned adults, true human beings? This is not a given. Traditionally this was the work of culture. Through the long labors of multiple initiations, individuals were gradually crafted into persons of substance and gravity. The process yielded someone more attuned to responsibilities than rights, more aware of multiple entanglements than entitlements. They were initiated into a vast sea of intimacies, with the village, star clusters and gnarled old oaks, the pool of ancestors, and the scented earth.

Through the sustained attention of culture, individuals were ripened into adults capable of sustaining culture: a marvelous symmetry.

We are meant to cross many thresholds in our lifetime, each a further embodiment of the soul's innate character. Yet many of us carry the uncomfortable thought that we are unsure of our place in the world, still anxious about our sense of value and our right to be here. The *unfinished business* of adolescence haunts us consciously and unconsciously and makes it hard to live into the larger arc of our lives.

Crossing the threshold from adolescence into adulthood requires an ordeal, a tempering of the individual that *begins* the process of ripening. There is no easy passage. Many traditional cultures escorted their youth into the world of adulthood and the sacred through an elaborate series of rituals. These rituals occurred in nature, in the holding space of forests and caves, savannahs, and bush. It was a space outside the ordinary world of the village, apart from the community, and often took place over many weeks and even months. It was a time of tempering the young ones with intense ritual ordeals that took them beyond their capacities to endure. Something died in the process. Something needed to die in the process. And something needed to come forward. Some new shape of identity that was wedded to the silt and slope of the land, which spoke the feathered and furred language of the creatures and the song of the dawn. This new identity was comingled with the holy topography. They became the same.

Underneath and holding up this initiatory process was a deep and abiding relationship to the wild world and the spirits of place. This passage was rooted in a nearly endless succession of generations that had come to learn the necessity of such a transition. The awareness for this is essentially universal: our souls must be shaped by a process of intense ritual encounter, communal reflection, and immersion in the natural and supranatural worlds. In other words, to become an adult, certain gateways needed to be crossed for that territory to be fully embedded within the person.

What we witness daily in the litany of injustices and exploitation of others and the world are the actions of uninitiated individuals. It is not difficult to see how questions of adequacy and inclusion are often portrayed in gross exaggerations of power and force. Nor is it a stretch to see how the persistent hunger in the unripened psyche of so many is at the heart of our violent consumption of the planet.

Initiation is an entrance into a place, a terrain. It is a courtship of a large dreaming animal. It is not an abstract ideal of psychological accomplishment, but an entrance into the specificity of locale, of geography, of rhizomes and crab thought, mercurial imaginings, moon cycles, and seasonal rhythms, with eyes that regard these as sacred. Through these intimacies, a grand landscape comes into vision: a world permeated with spirit, ancestors, community, cosmos, and the dreams of those yet to come.

Initiation, in its deepest traditional sense, was meant to keep the world alive. The purpose was not individual, but cosmological in scope. *It was never for the individual.* This is extremely hard for us to get our minds around, having been conditioned within a psychological tradition that fixates everything upon the "self." It is always about me and my growth! Here is the truth, however: *Initiation was an act of sacrifice on behalf of the greater circle of life into which the initiate is brought and to which they now hold allegiance.*

Can you feel your longing for just such a knowing?

At the same time, initiation profoundly affects us as individuals. It activates and authorizes the particular soul thread we came to offer the waiting world. Much like those seed pods that germinate only in the heat of fire, the soul seed we carry responds to the heat generated by initiation.

The soul is fully aware of the reciprocal relationship it has with the wild world, with the worlds of spirit and the ancestors. Soul recognizes the innate requirements for maintaining these connections. It was the role of mature individuals to honor our *place in the family of things* by conducting the rituals of gratitude and renewal that sustain our relations with the breathing, animate world. Initiation embeds in us a fundamental requirement of being human:

We are meant to feed Life in an ongoing way!

As we mature, we are asked to come into a more reciprocal relationship with the earth. We are called to develop the manners that help sustain the body of this exquisite world. Values such as respect, restraint, mutuality, reciprocity, gratitude, and courage help to fortify our ability to stand and protect what we love. We are here to participate in the ongoing creation, to offer our imagination, affection, and devotion to the sustaining of the world.

It is not difficult to see how modernity, with its emphasis on technology, speed, excessive consumption, and exaggerated individualism, has taken us far from these living practices. The central question is: How can we, once again, recognize the transforming cadence of initiation in a time of amnesia, a time in which the old forms have been abandoned?

The truth is *initiation is not optional*. Every one of us will be taken to the edge of our own ripening, pulled by the gravity of soul to engage the rigors of maturing us into something substantial. No one is exempt. Imagine if we could see the circumstances of our lives as the raw material necessary for the movement across the threshold into our adult lives. The times of loss, trauma, defeat, betrayal, and illness become the *prima materia*, the beginning matter, for undertaking the crossing into our more encompassing life. This could free us in radical ways. Seen from a mythic per-spective, these are the exact conditions that can help cook the soul and bring us closer to the mystery of our own singular incarna-tion. Rather than a commentary on our brokenness and worth-lessness, our wounds become the entry into the *unripened seeds of our initiation*. So much depends upon how we perceive what it is that is happening in our world. Taking a mythic view enables us to see our circumstances as necessary, even required, for the work of deep change to take place.

The need is clear: We must cultivate a robust collective of adults whose primary fealty is to the life-giving world upon which we depend. We must be able to feel our loyalties to watersheds, migratory pathways, marginalized communities, and the soul of the world. We must feel the bedrock of our aliveness and the real-ity of our wild and exuberant lives. Initiation tempers the soul, drawing out its hidden essence and calling forth the medicine we came to offer this stunning world. It is time to wake up!

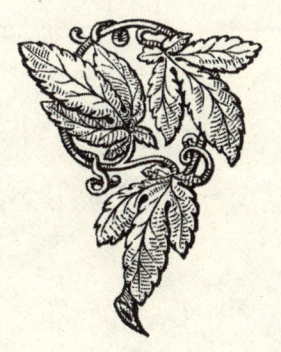

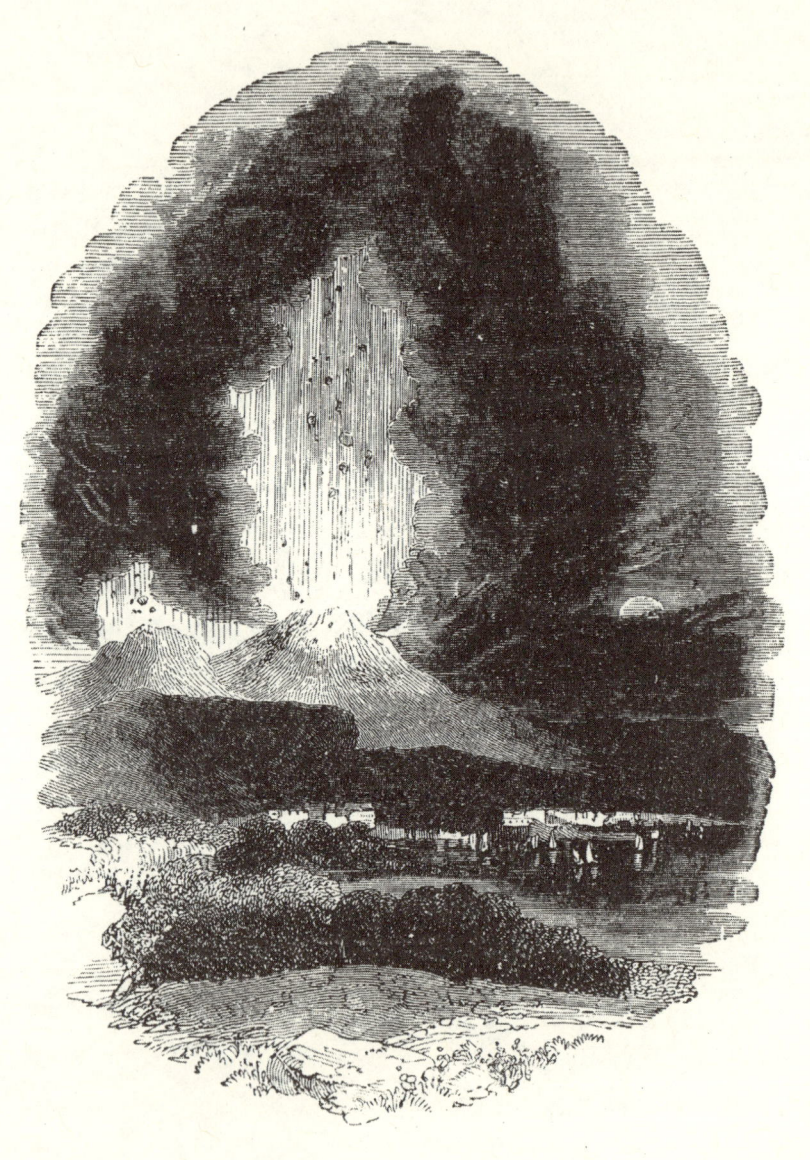

Three

Everything Is Burning

OVER THE PAST FEW YEARS, we have seen radical changes in the physical and psychic landscape of Northern California. The fires that began late on a Sunday night, in October of 2017, quickly engulfed homes and dreams, woodlands, and security. Many of us awoke in the middle of the night to the acrid smell of smoke, sensing that something was wrong. Only later, with the dawn light, were we able to see the extent of this disturbing truth. Since that time, wildfires have lit up landscapes around the planet. Much of Canada and Europe, Australia, and Russia have seen devastating fires consuming vast swaths of land and along with it, the lives of countless creatures.

Clearly, our souls have been shaken by this catastrophic event. Everyone has been affected, whether we lost a loved one, a home, a beloved pet, our place of employment, a trail that we cherished, or simply our sense of faith in the ordinary assurances of daily life. No one in our community has been spared the sorrows that have fallen upon us like ash. We are living in a collective field of sorrows that will take a long, long time to metabolize. In the years that have followed, the presence of wildfires has become constant.

In some northern European cultures, the season of grieving the loss of someone close was known as a period of *living in the ashes*. This extended time was an era of descent, a movement into the underworld where the bitter tincture of grief was meant to be churned and metabolized into medicine for the community. It was a sacred time, a time out of time, in which the primary work was digesting sorrow. We have felt and seen the swirl of ash in the air. We are all being asked to do the sacred work of transmuting loss into wisdom.

How are we to respond when life confronts us with overwhelming circumstances? How can we hold all we are feeling when the source of the feelings is far beyond our ability to control? How do we recalibrate our inner lives to further the healing reflex of the psyche in times of trauma? Here are a few offerings for a medicine kit for tending our souls during traumatic times. And who isn't living in traumatic times?

1. **Practice self-compassion.** During periods of stress, we often fall back on old patterns of relating to ourselves and the world. We can be harsh and critical, withholding, and brittle, especially with ourselves. Self-compassion offers us the opportunity to hold what is vulnerable with kindness and tenderness, allowing these places to remain soft and open. Times of great uncertainty call for a level of generosity to ourselves that helps to offset the effects of trauma that can often envelop our emotional bodies. This must be our first and primary intention: to hold all that we are experiencing with compassion; to offer a safe place for our fears and grief to land.

   Self-compassion is the foundation for befriending our lives. It is the great work of the heart to behold our life as eminently worthy of compassion and love. We will not figure our way through this maze of grief and suffering. We must, instead, learn to turn toward our sorrows with kindness, tenderness, and affection. Lean in. Offer love, a touch of affection. Nothing ever heals in an atmosphere of judgment or criticism. We contract and get small under such conditions. We open and soften only when the space around us invites revelation and connection.

A working definition of self-compassion is that it is the *internalized village*. Imagine how a dear friend would respond to your pain and suffering, fear, and grief when they arise. Whereas we can be impatient and judgmental about our inner states, a good friend would offer us a holding space big enough to be with what it is we are experiencing and touch it with mercy. We are all worthy of compassion, and when we can turn toward our pain or grief with kindness, we open our hearts and grant the conditions necessary for healing.

2. **Turn toward the feelings.** There is no bypass or strategy of avoidance that can help resolve the difficult emotions we will encounter. Turning toward our suffering is essential. We must not only endure our times of pain and sorrow, hoping to get to the far shore of them, but we must also actively engage them and feel them fully. This move takes great courage. It is hard to open ourselves up to the painful emotions that await us without an adequate level of compassion and support.

   There is a premise in the alchemical tradition that says we must keep the materials warm for them to ripen in the vessel. If we do not, our sorrows and fears will harden and congeal, making movement impossible. When we hold these challenging emotions with affection, concern, compassion, and interest, they stay flexible and fluid, capable of change. We keep them warm by holding a steady vigil with these difficult guests and not turning away and neglecting what these pieces of our soul life need from us.

When we offer this kind of devotion, our sorrows and fears will change. As the poet Rilke reminds us, "No feeling is final."[7]

To feel it fully, however, we require the arms and hearts of others, tethering us to a wider circle of belonging. The weight of grief and suffering that we are facing is more than we can hold in isolation. Be willing to share what has been gathered in your heart with another. Call three or four friends together and share the communal cup of loss that we are all feeling in this uncertain time. Be mindful of how much conditioning we have received that tells us to go it alone; to not need anyone or bother anyone else with our struggles. Challenge those thoughts. "This is," as one of my teachers said, "the solitary journey we cannot do alone."[8] Coming into the company of others, human and more-than-human, reassures us and adds to the internal feeling of safety.

3. **Be astonished by beauty.** Trauma has a profound impact on our feelings of aliveness, often generating a state of numbness or anesthesia. This state protects us for a time from having to encounter the raw, searing emotions that often accompany trauma, but it also dulls our sensual engagement with all that surrounds us. At some point, we will be required to meet the painful emotions and the sediment of sorrows that have accumulated around us. Beauty's allure helps to open the full aperture of the heart. Sorrow and beauty side by side. The soul has a fundamental need for encounters with beauty. Beauty is a central source of nourishment that continually renews our sense of vitality and awe.

Beauty calls us outward into the world. It quickens the senses, awakens the heart, and pulls us deeper into intimacy with the folds of the world. The poet Robinson Jeffers said our love was meant to fall outward into the astonishingly beautiful world that surrounds us. Immerse yourself in beauty. Bring flowers into whatever space you occupy, along with fragrances that enchant and soothe. Play music that touches your heart and sing along. Read the poetry of Akhmatova, Dickinson, Machado, and Neruda. As Rumi said, "Let the beauty we love be what we do."[9] The felt encounter with beauty increases our sense of ease, connection, and re-regulation.

4. **Have patience.** Healing from trauma takes time. Patience offers a courtesy to the vulnerable pieces of soul life that have been splintered by the presence of trauma. Knitting a bone takes time. Mending the soul takes even longer. Be patient with your process. There is deep wisdom in the soul that knows the value of going slowly. Pause for a few moments a day, under the stars, beneath the generous shade of an old oak, with a cup of tea. Stepping out of the manic pace of modern culture is essential to regain our footing in the world of soul. Patience is a discipline, a practice that offers assurance to the places of vulnerability and a ground for absorbing the benefits of our efforts.

Patience creates a state of spaciousness where the deeper rhythms of the soul can reemerge. Patience also invites a creative emptiness where the unimagined can arise. We are not the authors of our healing. Our task is to generate a space of receptivity to dreams, images, insights, intuitions, and inspirations, all through the hospitality of patience.

The Buddha said in one of his sermons, "Everything is burning."[10] In these extreme times, the truth of impermanence strikes at the very heart of our lives. Everything we hold dear—loved ones, homes, photos of family and ancestors, objects that hold a sense of the sacred—can all be gone in a flash. What remains are the bonds of love and friendship. What we witnessed during the smoke-filled days following the onset of the fires were acts of kindness, gestures of generosity, and a recognition that our lives are mutually entangled with one another. May this spirit endure. May we find the courage we need to keep our hearts open to one another and to this wild, fragrant earth. Stay safe. Become a house of belonging.

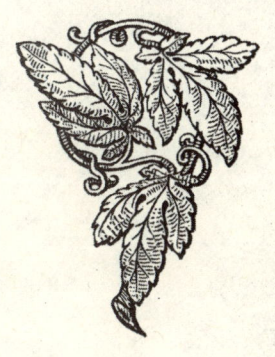

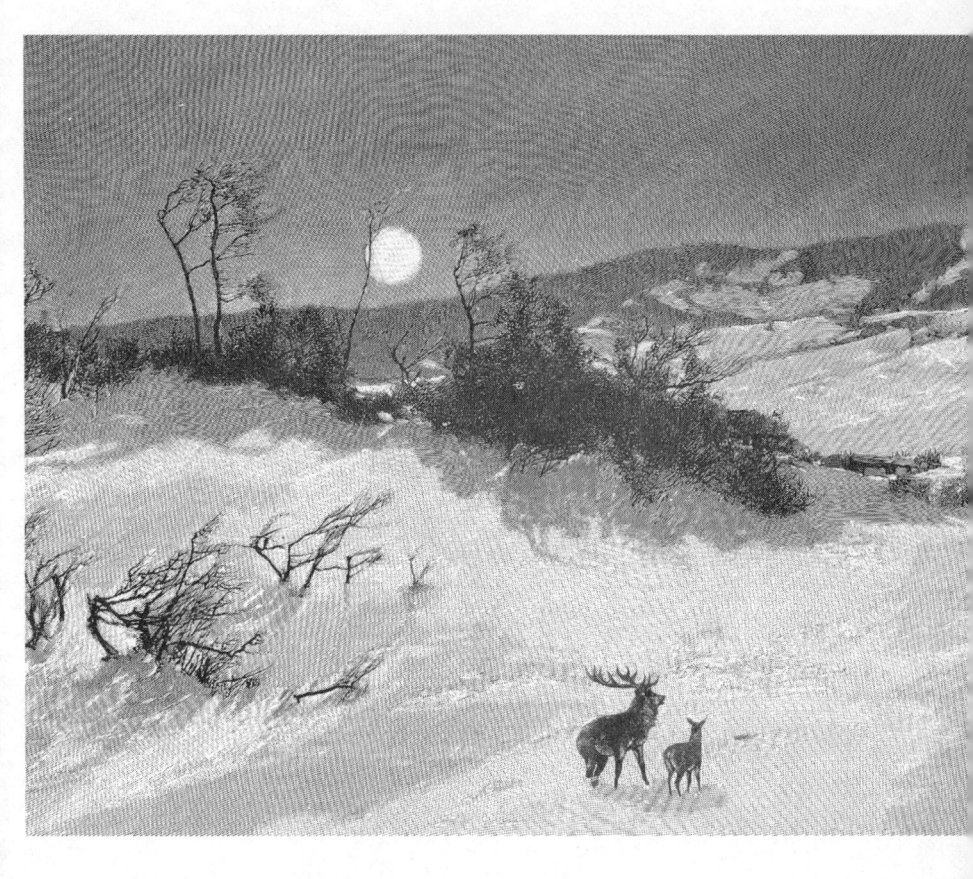

Four

An Apprenticeship with Sorrow

This night will pass, then we have work to do.[11]
—RUMI

GRIEF AND LOSS TOUCH US ALL, arriving at our door in many ways. They come swirling on the winds of divorce, upon the death of someone dear, or as an illness that alters the course of a life. For many of us, grief is tied intimately to the ravages we witness daily to watersheds and forests, the extinction of species, the collapse of democracy, and the fading of civilization. Left unattended, these sorrows can seep underground, shadowing our days. It is our unexpressed sorrows, the congested stories of loss, that, when left untouched, block our access to the vitality of the soul. To be able to freely move in and out of the soul's inner chambers, we must first clear the way. This requires finding meaningful ways to speak of sorrow. It requires that we take up an *apprenticeship with sorrow*. Learning to welcome, hold, and metabolize sorrow is the work of a lifetime.

Our apprenticeship begins when we come to understand that grief is ever-present in our lives. This is a difficult realization, but one that has the opportunity of opening our hearts to a deeper love for our singular life and for the windswept world of which we are a part. We begin with the simple gesture of picking up the shards of grief that lie littered on the floor of our house.

Nothing special. Nothing heroic. Not unlike the young novices entering their apprenticeship with the master teacher, we begin humbly, sweeping the shavings, mixing the pigments, cleaning the brushes, and tending the fires. We begin the process by building our capacity to hold sorrow in the womb of the heart. Through this practice, we become able to welcome the pervasive and encompassing presence of grief.

> *Grief works us in profound ways, reshaping us moment by moment*
> *in the heat of loss. We are also asked to work grief and to*
> *take up our apprenticeship with fidelity and love.*

It takes tremendous psychic strength to engage the wild images, searing emotions, chaotic dreams, grief-stained memories, and visceral sensations that arise in times of deep grief. We must build soul muscle to meet these times with anything resembling affection. *The apprenticeship is long.*

Grief is more than an emotion; it is also a *core faculty of being human*. It is a skill that must be developed, or we will find ourselves migrating to the margins of our lives in hopes of avoiding the inevitable entanglements with loss. It is through the rites of grief that we are ripened as human beings. Grief brings gravity and depth into our world. We possess the profound capacity to metabolize sorrow into something medicinal for our soul and the soul of the community. The skill of grieving well enables us to become *current*—to live in the present moment and be available to the electricity of life. We gradually turn our attention to what is here, now, and pay less attention to our need to repair history. We remember we are more verb than noun, more a jumpy rhythm, a wild song, a fluid leap than a fixed thing in space. As Spanish poet Jaime Gil de Biedma said, "I believed I wanted to be a poet, but deep down I just wanted to be a poem."[12]

I find the idea of apprenticeship helpful. Rather than something acquired quickly and with minimal effort, an apprenticeship conveys a prolonged period of study and immersion, an extended conversation with the materials of loss, its leaden weight and intense emotions. There are multiple elements in our apprenticeship with sorrow. The first is coming to understand the need to develop *right relationship* with grief, not pushing it away or drowning in it. We tend to experience grief in one or the other of these binary postures. Coming to know sorrow as a companion helps to ease our fear and offers us the opportunity to come into a more ongoing and abiding connection with this inevitable presence in our lives.

Secondly, we are asked to cultivate a *practice* of some sort to offer ballast when the sea tide of sorrow rises in our world. A practice steadies us, helps us to remain present to work the material that is there. Our apprenticeship is a sustained practice in the art of vesseling,* learning how to hold, contain, separate, and warm the materials of loss and sorrow. Any practice, from meditation to prayer, yoga to writing, helps us to keep the grief fluid and able to keep moving.

The third layer in our apprenticeship concerns our ability to *stay present in the adult* when working with the movements of sorrow in our world. Only the adult can work with grief. Only the adult has the spaciousness and skill to hold and engage sorrow's tangled edges. This requires us to recognize who carries the central story around grief. Frequently it is a child state that is the default response to grief. This aspect in our interior life does not possess the capacity to digest the difficult and often bitter tincture of sorrow. Learning how to migrate this into the adult's hands is central to our apprenticeship.[13]

---

* See chapter 8, "The Art of Vesseling."

Silence and solitude form the next layer in our apprenticeship. Much of our encounter with loss and sorrow will be alone. Deepening a relationship with silence and solitude is essential in fostering an internal state that is able to be with our times of grief in a generative way. Silence is a form of hospitality to what is most tender in us. It offers a courtesy of attention and witnessing that is often lacking in our cultural attitudes of getting beyond our grief as soon as possible. Solitude is a deep bow to the soul's need for time alone in which to bring a patient affection for these raw and vulnerable emotions.

The next element in our work with grief is *self-compassion*. I wrote in *The Wild Edge of Sorrow* that grief work opens the pathway to compassion for others. What I didn't say was that self-compassion is required for us to open ourselves to our own losses. Self-compassion is not an event but an ongoing practice, a ritual of remembering the simple truth that we need to respond to our experiences of loss with warmth and kindness, a soft and caring heart. There is no healing path that does not course through the territory of self-compassion.

Our final element is *remembering our wild entanglement with all our relations*. We cannot face the sorrows of the world or our own personal encounters with loss in isolation. We need to feed a robust companionship with the wider world, with the cosmos itself. Our apprenticeship is rooted in this extended sense of kinship with the surrounding watersheds, the microbes and root structures, the clouds and star clusters. When we remember these filaments of relationship with all that is, we are fortified and potent enough to turn into the heat of all that is.

This apprenticeship is, at heart, about the shaping of elders:
the ones capable of meeting the pain and suffering of the
world with a dignified and robust bearing.

After years of walking alongside grief, working with its difficult cargo, we gradually come to see how we have been reshaped by this companionship. We see how we have cultivated a greater interior space to hold more of what life brings to us. What slowly emerges from this long apprenticeship, this vigil with sorrow, is a spaciousness capable of holding it all—the beauty and the loss, the despair and the yearning, the fear and the love. We become immense: *The apprenticeship is patiently crafting an elder*.

After years of holding steady with sorrow, a distillation of wisdom occurs. We develop a capacity to see in the darkness and find there, in the depths of it all, something holy, something eternal. We touch the indwelling sacredness of the life we inhabit, digesting bitterness and returning with a determination to feed the community. We become a hive of imagination, dispensing what we have gathered over this extended education of the heart. What was learned was not meant for us alone but was meant to be tossed like a seed into a fertile mind, a waiting community, a hungry culture.

Elders are a composite of contradictions: fierce and forgiving, joyful and melancholy, intense and spacious, solitary and communal. They have been seasoned by a long fidelity to love and loss. We become elders by accepting life on life's terms, gradually relinquishing the fight to have it fit our expectations. An elder has no quarrel with the ways of the world. Initiated through many years of loss, they have come to know that life is hard, riddled with failures, betrayals, and deaths. They have made peace with the imperfections that are inherent in life. The wounds and losses they encounter become the material with which to shape a life of meaning, humor, joy, depth, and beauty. They do not push away suffering, nor wish to be exempt from the inevitable losses that come. They know the futility of such a wish. This acceptance, in turn, frees them to radically receive the stunning elegance of the world.

Ultimately, an elder is a storehouse of living memory, a carrier of wisdom. Elders are the voice that rises on behalf of the commons, at times fiery, at times beseeching. They live simultaneously outside culture and as its greatest protectors, becoming wily dispensers of love and blessings. They offer a resounding "yes" to the generations that follow them. That is their legacy and gift.

When the season is right, when we have been tempered sufficiently by the heat of life, we are asked to accept the mantle of elderhood as the most ordinary of things. Nothing special about it. It is ordinary to know loss and sorrow, to be taken below the surface of life and be reshaped by the currents of grief. It is ordinary to be deepened by the draw of sorrow and its intense wash, clearing away old debris and outdated strategies. It is ordinary to feel the aperture of the heart open because of our intimacy with grief. No longer compelled by the allure of being special, we are free to take our place in the world, casting blessings by the simple offer of our presence, seasoned by sorrow.

This is how elders are crafted: tempered between the heat of loss and the weight of loving this world.

We are all preparing for our own disappearance, our one last breath. It is difficult to pick up this thread and hold it in our hands. Each of us is fated to leave this shining world, to slip off this elegant coat of skin, to release our stories to the wind, and to return our bones to the earth. Saying goodbye, however, is neither easy nor something we give much thought to in our daily lives.

How do we say goodbye? How do we acknowledge all that has held beauty and value in our lives—those we love, those who touched our lives with kindness, those whose shelter allowed us to extend ourselves into the world? How do we let go of sunsets and making love, pomegranates, and walks on the bluff? And yet, we must. We must release the entire fantastic world with one last breath. We will all fall into the Mystery. We are most alive at the threshold of loss and revelation.

Our fidelity to our apprenticeship with sorrow is key to keeping our souls open and engaged with the living world and offering our unique gifts to the community. Being able to metabolize grief into medicine is to be used well by the soul of the world.

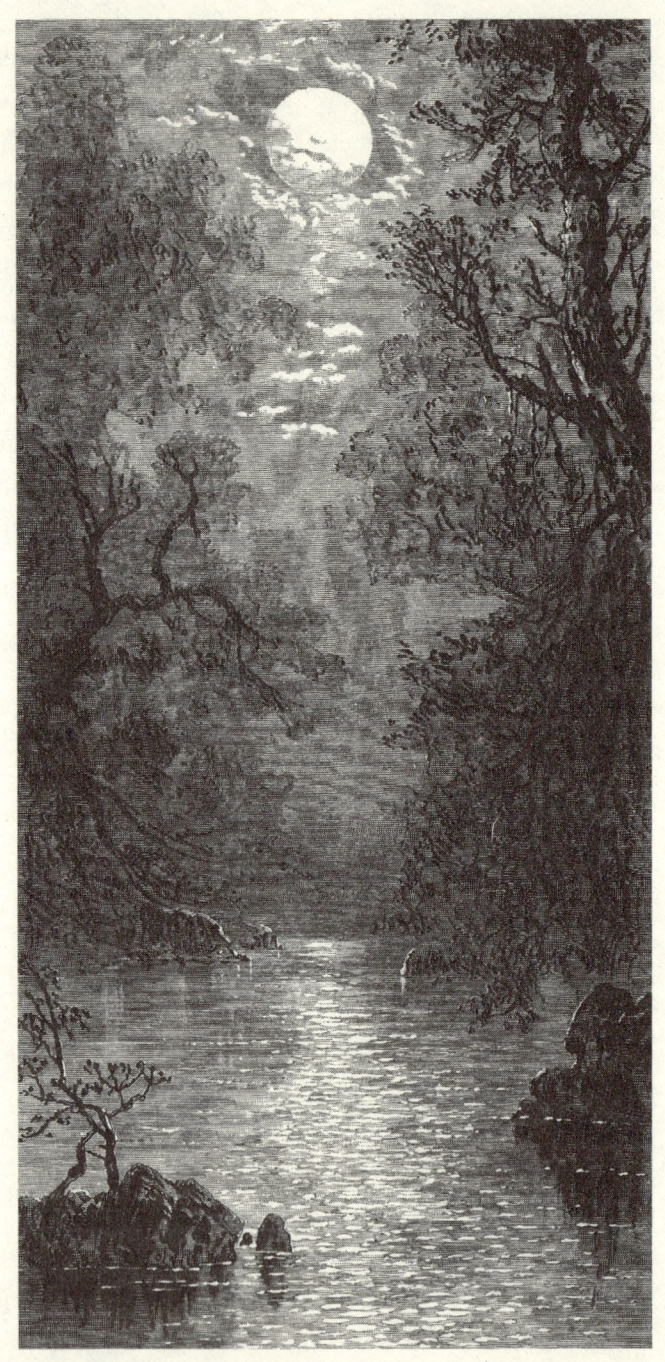

Five

Baptized in Dark Waters

I have faith in nights.[14]

—RAINER MARIA RILKE

THERE ARE TIMES, more akin to seasons, when we are brought down into the terrain of shadows. These times are not caused by something happening in our daylit world, nor by history or genetic inheritance. We are required to periodically surrender and meander in the vast uncharted terrain of the underworld. These are times initiated by soul. Most of us will have times like this. They will descend upon us, as they say, "out of the blue." In truth, it is more blue bending toward black.

Dante's famous lyric poem, *The Divine Comedy*, begins memorably with the lines

In the middle of the road of my life, I awoke in a
dark wood, where the true way was wholly lost.[15]

His words are oddly reassuring, reminding us that this does happen to most everyone. Sometimes we awake in a dark wood, where the way is wholly lost. His words simultaneously unsettle us as they confirm that these times leave us feeling lost. It seems we are not fully in charge of our interior lives. We are required to periodically descend and enter the vast unknown territory of the underworld.

In alchemy, these seasonal migrations were called times in the *nigredo*, or the blackening. It is helpful to see this as an inevitable and necessary time, a time of shedding and letting go, of sitting close to the furnace of death as it cooks away all that is spent and no longer serving life. Our time in the *nigredo* is a period of dissolution. Old patterns and perceptions, old, outworn identities begin to dissolve as we are unmade. Things fall apart. There is an unraveling, an emptying of hope, and an undermining of our great heroic enterprise to be in control and rise above our suffering. We are taken down to the ground and asked, as psychotherapist Jennifer Welwood said, to "dance the wild dance of no hope!"[16]

Anyone who has ever been escorted into the underworld knows full well how uncharted this place feels. We are without fixed stars, known destinations, familiar markers, or guideposts. The *nigredo* was called the "subtle dissolver" in alchemy and was viewed as a necessary element in the great work of creating the *philosopher's stone*. The work could commence through the attainment of the *nigredo*. Only when the familiar structures were eroded was it possible for something new to arise. It is difficult for us to see our time in the underworld as something required for the deepening of our soul life. One major challenge to this understanding is that we are highly conditioned to strive for the light, rise above everything, and overcome every obstacle. Not so when soul pulls us downward.

The *nigredo* often initiates an eclipse of the familiar self. We feel a thinning, a loosening of our fixed sense of identity. Our progressive fantasies are confounded by the pull of the *nigredo*. The blue moods—irritated, sullen, heavy, sad—insult our fictions of progress and having it all together. The summons is a call to a more intimate and collaborative relationship with the darkness that accompanies soul.

We meet a different self in this grotto of darkness, someone closer to the dream world and comfortable in shadowed places. This one knows about melancholy and has not been swept up in the pursuit of the light. We need to know this other one who is more kindred with the nature of shimmering moonlight and soul than the brilliant sunlight of consciousness. This self sees through the layers of conditioning we all endure that oppress and domesticate. This one expresses something true and alive whether through the complex rhythms of the blues, in shades of nuanced speech, or in the tender intimacy of vulnerability. This other is inclined to silence, the night sky, the poetry of Neruda and Machado, and the friendship of solitude.

When we find ourselves walking through the ink-black night of the underworld, we quickly begin looking for the exit door. The old myths and the teachings of alchemy suggest we take a different direction. The work, they say, is to move closer to the heart of the darkness. The alchemists said it clearly: The work is to make the black "blacker than black," the "color of a raven's head."

Not exactly the news we were hoping for.

Our attempts to leave the loom of night too soon, however, may deprive us of the work being done in the dark, often without our awareness. Much happens in this underground domain outside of our attention and control. What is missing is our engagement with the black threads of soul. This is a time of faith, but not necessarily one of hope. Faith that this is a place of value, a terrain filled with richness—not unlike the black earth—something capable of nourishing new tremulous pieces of soul into life. Coming to understand that much happens outside of our conscious interventions is freeing and adds to our faith in the capacities of soul to take us where we need to go in these unexpected times of descent.

Our sojourn in the darkness, while difficult and often painful, is also a time of alteration and change. The process of change, however, is not one of addition and growth but one of letting go, decay, subtraction, and death, what the alchemists called *putre-factio*. It is a *via negativa*, a road of negation. Like nature, it has a returning rhythm of slow movements or stillness, repetitive thoughts and feelings, and memories that arise repeatedly. We come to see that this season is necessary for any spring to unfold. With a measure of fidelity to the work, this season of uncertainty is gradually digested into something dense and full. When we are able to carry these times with faithfulness, it yields a gravitas, a tincture of wisdom for the waiting village.

Archetypal psychologist Stanton Marlan writes powerfully about the value of the descent. In his book *The Black Sun: The Alchemy and Art of Darkness*, Marlan states, "Blackness is not a stage to be bypassed once and for all, but a necessary component of psychological life. Blackness has a purpose: It teaches endurance, warns, dissolves attachments, and sophisticates the eye so that we may not only see blackness but actually see by means of it."[17] The darkness invites a different mode of seeing, ripened by the seasonality of our times in the *nigredo*. And isn't this what happens when we engage our grief, our vulnerability: a new landscape slowly appears?

Our time in the underworld brings us close to sorrow. Our grief carries love in it; love darkened by the loss of friends, homes, marshes, marriages, children, animals, and dreams. It is this mode of love that leads us toward the black tones of *duende*, a fierce love—musty, gritty, and suffused with powdered glass. We weep tears of darkness, gripped by what is calling us close to the earth. *Duende* is a wild, vital energy, and when it touches us, as it often does when sorrow's fingers caress the soul, we feel strangely unsettled, as though something in our underground world has been violently shaken. We feel a strange mixture of immobility—weighed down by the sediments of grief—and activation in the deep cavern of soul when *duende* moves us. *Duende* asks for movement, for some form of expression that honors the depth of feeling that is present. It rises through the soles of our feet, carrying the black earth into our bodies aching for full voice.

The great Spanish poet and eloquent writer on *duende*, Federico García Lorca, wrote that whoever is touched by *duende* is "baptized in dark waters."[18] This is a potent image that intimates that these are holy waters that arise when we find ourselves moving through the terrain of the underworld. This baptism is one in which we are washed by the waters of our own tears, the very salt of the soul, and united with the realm of the sacred. It is no wonder that we often return changed and ripened from our time in the arms of grief. "The duende's arrival," Lorca says, "always means a radical change in forms."[19]

It may be that the "most important secrets hide in the shadows,"[20] as Buddhist teacher Joan Halifax writes. To find them, we must be willing to enter the darkness and discover what is waiting there to be brought back to the hungry world. Dive deep!

> **REFLECTION QUESTION:**   Recall a time when you found yourself in unexplained darkness: a mood that settled upon you for an extended period that crowded out the light. Sit with this memory, not so much to figure it out, what it meant, but more, what effect did this time have upon you? What was asked of you in this time of shadows? Write for fifteen minutes.

PART II

&

Care of the Soul

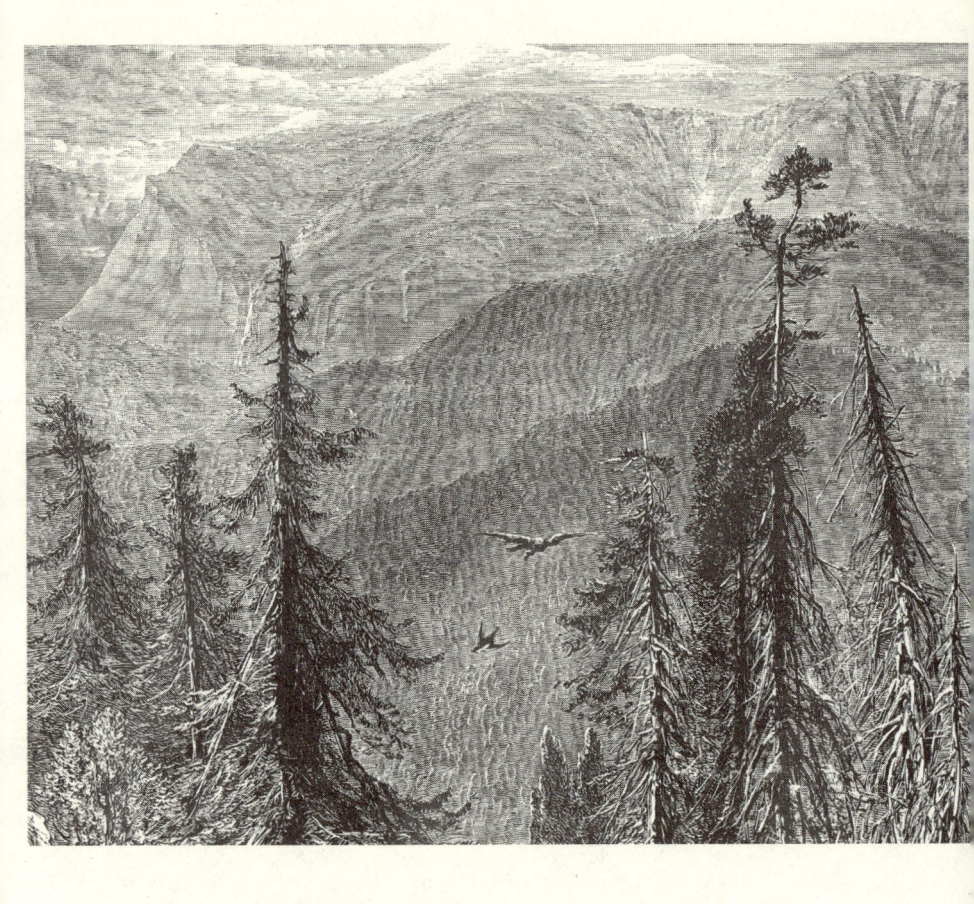

Six

The Grandeur of the Soul

DURING THE RENAISSANCE, when the world still possessed a sense of enchantment, when animals and the dreaming Earth spoke and were worthy of our attention, poets and philosophers conjured an image to depict the grandeur of the soul. What they came upon was the night sky. That is how vast and mysterious we are. That is how unfathomable and beautiful we are. Pause and think about this. Breathe it into yourself. This is our true inheritance: the wild, undulating majesty of the soul. When we let this larger reality fall upon us, we drift into the grand expanse of the soul. This is what we long for, and it is nested in the heart of our ancestral memory. Soul as root, as well as heartbeat, the perennial ground that binds the human and the more-than-human worlds together.

The emphasis in our time, however, is upon the self. The "me" that we most often identify with inside our definitions. It is curious that we often feel small and isolated when embedded solely in this identity. That may be because the self is experienced as insular, interior, segregated, and partitioned off from others in the world. Matters of boundaries and individuation abound. Specialness, mastery, and self-improvement flood the psychological landscape. And yet, for all the offers of psychological development, the feelings of separation still linger. We have forgotten the grandeur of the soul, our innate inheritance, and have been reduced to trying to keep ourselves afloat in the boat of self.

I am not denying the presence of a self, an identity that gives each of us a bearing in the world. What I am calling our attention to is that without soul, the self remains marooned in its isolated hut of interiority. It is the soul that leads us into the wild interplay *between* self and world, between self and ancestors, the Dream-time and spirit, and the profusion of images arising continuously from the psyche. Soul is there, betwixt and between, eliciting connections and intimacies. We fall *into* the world via the soul's erotic desire for this sensuous life.

Soul offers continual intimations of belonging. And isn't that what we need in these times—a sense of belonging that is entangled with melting glaciers, cedar waxwings, the cries of families separated at borders, and whispers shared deep in the night between lovers? To step into the domain of soul is to enter a rich and vibrant terrain punctuated with images and eruptions of affection. It is to step across a threshold and find ourselves enraptured by the *deep story* of the soul displayed in myths, metaphors, and mystery.

Soul is a shapeshifter, wearing many coats. Whereas the self prefers definitions and structure, soul is too rambunctious to be contained in one simple story, particularly our biographical narrative. That is, in part, why there are so many variations of fairy tales and myths. Soul requires a multitude of ways to express its full nature. The extensive array of images found in these wisdom tales reminds us that the ground of our being is wide and deep. We are part wind, part track of moonlight on water, part dreaming coyote, part slumbering bear. To attend to these wider strands of soul life binds us with the dreaming Earth, the soul of the world. Loneliness abates and the edges of our identity thin and become permeable. We remember our expanded selves and find ourselves at home.

When we look up into the bowl of night and take in the exquisite beauty of the stars, we are catching a glimpse of the eternal and a mirror of our own immense lives. We have been gifted with this stunning life, and along with this comes an innate responsibility to live it fully. And since the soul is at home with all the manifestations of this world, from joy to sorrow, despair to astonishment, and everything in between, let us risk seeing ourselves as part of the grandeur of the soul.

Soul Work

Take some time one of these nights and lie out under the canopy of stars. Let your imagination go and let it invite you into a reverie that suggests that what you are seeing is also a reflection of your own vastness. What if that is true? What if you, as Walt Whitman suggests, are large and contain multitudes? How might you walk differently in the world? How would your story of yourself change to account for the larger and wider sense of identity? Write about this for fifteen minutes or share your reflections with a friend.

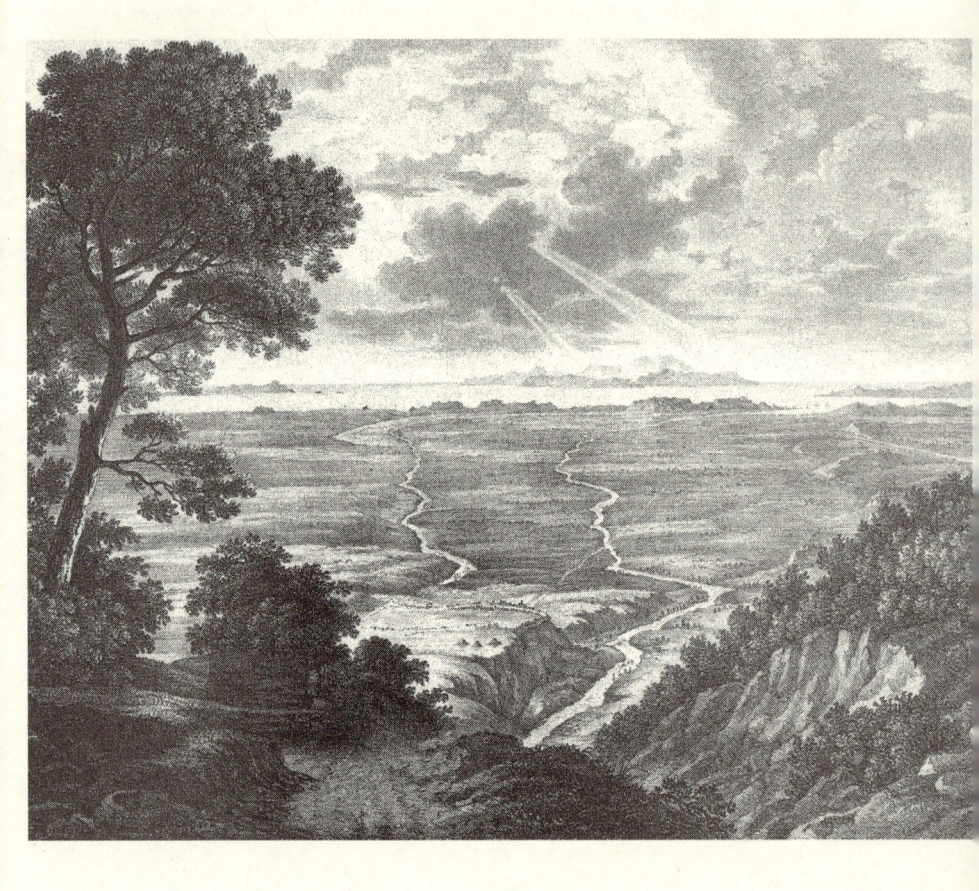

Seven

The Reverence of Approach

SEVERAL YEARS AGO, I came across a passage by the Irish poet and philosopher John O'Donohue. His words profoundly impacted my thoughts and have become somewhat of an interior anthem in my life. In his book *Beauty: The Invisible Embrace*, O'Donohue writes, "What you encounter, recognize or discover depends to a large degree on the quality of your approach. . . . When we approach with reverence, great things decide to approach us."[21]

This passage is rich with implications. As I have sat with it over the years and offered it to others in my therapy work and in workshop settings, I have continually seen its wisdom and value. For example, when we turn our attention to the inner world, we frequently do so with an eye toward evaluation and critique. We look for flaws and defects, casting about for evidence of failure. This gaze is harsh and causes the soul to retreat. Over forty years in my psychotherapy practice, I have never seen anything open or change in an atmosphere of judgment. An approach of reverence, on the other hand, is foundational to a life imbued with soul. From this way of seeing, we recognize that everything possesses a measure of the sacred, including our sorrows and pain. How we approach our inner life profoundly affects what comes to us in return.

What we encounter, recognize, or discover depends on the quality of our approach. An approach of reverence invites revelation.

To pause and reflect on this can make all the difference between living in a cold, detached world, populated primarily by judgments and cynicism, and living in a world suffused with intimacy and offers of communion. When our approach is one of reverence, we find ourselves falling into a deeper embrace with all that is open to encounter, both internally and in the surrounding, breathing world. If we approach superficially, or from a perspective of what can we get out of this exchange, then the encounter will be limited, what we recognize will be thin, and what we discover will be nothing at all. We will simply be meeting our own well-rehearsed stories in the moment.

There is an intimation in O'Donohue's passage: He tells us that great things will approach us when we practice the etiquette of reverence. It is as if the aperture of our perception widens when we bring reverence to bear. We become able to recognize the holiness that exists in the moment, as I experienced this morning on my drive to work. As I came around a bend, winding through vineyards and meadows, the mist was threading its way at the base of the hills and in that glimpse, something great approached me. I was moved by the vista, brought to tears through the intimacy shared between my heart and the world.

An approach of reverence establishes a foundation ripe for amazement. We are readied for surprise and awe by a posture of reverence. It is a stance of humility, recognizing that the otherness that surrounds us—that infuses the world—is vast and powerful and yet curiously open for connection. An approach of reverence invites the mystery of an encounter where two solitudes meet and become entangled, creating a *third body*, an intimacy born of affection. All true intimacy requires an approach of reverence, deep regard, and an *unknowing* of who or what we are meeting. It is our bow honoring the exchange.

O'Donohue cautions us, however, that "the rushed heart and arrogant mind lack the gentleness and patience to enter that embrace."[22] We must be able to step out of the frantic and breathless pace that consumes much of our days. Reverence requires a rhythm akin to prayer. We are asked to slow down and rest in the space of silence and deep listening. There is a saying in the Zen tradition: "Not-knowing is most intimate." When we suspend our preconceptions and static stories of who we are, or who our wife, husband, or partner is; when we let go of our predetermined expectations of how it all should be, then we come into a place of reverence, of deep respect; and the freshness of the encounter is once again available to us. When we pause and notice, we are free to drink in the delicious thickness of the moment and all that it offers.

Reverence, rather than expectation or entitlement, acknowledges we live in a gifting cosmos and that we honor creation by singing praises. As the poet Rilke said, "To praise is the whole thing! A man who can praise / comes toward us like ore out of the silences / of rock."[23] Reverence acknowledges that what we are seeing or seeking is holy; that we depend utterly on this world to breathe and to dream.

We are designed for encounter; our senses are rivers of connection in a continuous exchange with the world around us. How deeply we experience this encounter, what we come to recognize and discover, is a question of presence, of reverence.

Soul Work

INNER WORK: Experiment with reverence over the coming days. Be mindful of how you approach your inner world. Is it characterized by criticism and judgment? Imagine coming to your experience with reverence, especially around your more vulnerable states like fear or grief. Notice the difference when you come to your experience with reverence. Take ten minutes and write about your experience.

OUTER WORK: Take a walk and let something call to your attention—a tree, a rose, a budding maple, an old barn. Soften your gaze and let the qualities of reverence fill your being. Simply notice what takes shape between the two of you. Allow the connection to come full and then offer your gratitude for the encounter. Remember, everything is open to conversation. Take ten minutes and write about your experience.

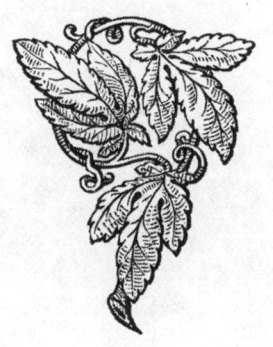

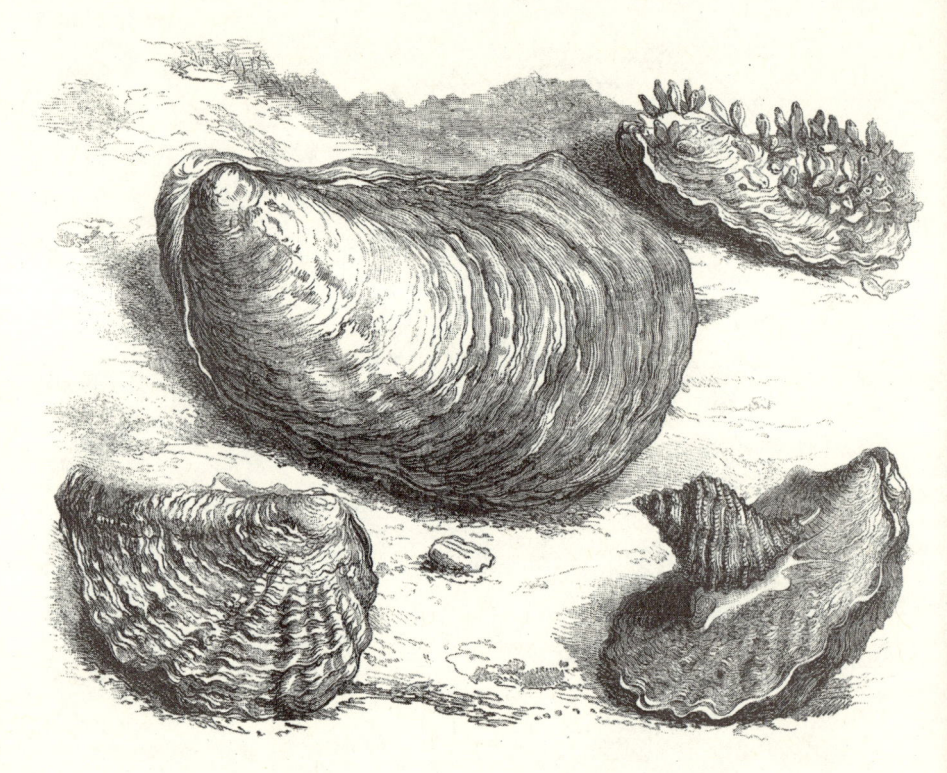

Eight

The Art of Vesseling

If God had not given us a vessel, His other gifts
would have been to no avail.[24]
—ALBERTUS MAGNUS

THE IDEA OF THE VESSEL is one frequently referenced in spiritual traditions and in the work of therapy. The idea suggests that deep psychic work requires a holding space, a secure container, within which the work of change can take place. When grief arises, in any one of its many shapes, it asks to be held by us, carried close to the heart, and nourished by our affection. We are asked to slowly build a vessel spacious enough to contain all the wild movements of a soul in grief. Grief, as we know, pulls us into another terrain, shadowed and dense, littered with the debris of loss. Uncontained, the swell of sorrow can overflow, and we can be carried away in a wash of grief. We need a space strong enough to contain the associated threads that accompany grief. It must be able to hold bitterness, remorse, and heartache so intense that we know for sure we will not survive. It must be able to hold cries of despair and hopelessness, long stretches of emptiness, and the writhing pains of betrayal. The vessel must be strong.

Grief activates the move to build the vessel. We intuitively know that what is moving in the hallways of the soul requires our attention, time, and devotion. These very acts are what generate the vessel. The vessel is created by work that takes place both within and without. It is shaped by how we hold what is present in our lives and it is enriched by how we are held by the surrounding field of friendships and the world. The inner work is one of noticing and responding to the push and pull of sorrow. It is about a courtship with lamentation, welcoming the many moods, old memories, and dreams that repeatedly arise. The inner work invokes silence and solitude as places of hospitality for our suffering hearts. The outer work takes on the wisdom of sharing wisely what is moving in us with those who can receive what it is we are expressing without judgment or advice.

Inner and outer overlap, strengthening the vessel, enabling us to do the demanding work of ripening grief into something dense and fortifying. We are asked to not solely endure our times of grief but to actively engage the materials, the weighty lead of loss, the black pitch of regrets, the salt mines of old wounds, and cook them slowly into a rich substance. The offer of attention keeps the material in the vessel warmed. Grief, left unattended, turns cold, hardens, and congeals. In this state of neglect, there is no possibility of movement. We become a chronic carrier of grief, permafrost forming in our subterranean lives. We are deadened and dulled when grief remains untended. We are asked to bring our warmth to the material and slowly allow it to cook. This is the work of alchemy.

The work of the vessel is both to contain and
to further the material.

Only what is held can flower. Only what is contained
can become something more than how it began.

The sorrows we encounter work their effects on us if we can engage the grief in a meaningful way. Held in a vessel of our making, shaped by vigilance and compassion, our grief is slowly ripened into a tincture of medicine for the waiting community.

Containment enables us to engage in the difficult dialogue between ourselves and the core of the melancholy, which would otherwise be dismissed by our enterprising mind, which has no time for such conversations. And yet, it is here, in the flux of loss and sorrow, that soul is deepened. Here, in the valley of grief, is where the character of soul is shaped.

Central to the work of alchemy was the image of the vessel. As one noted alchemist, Albertus Magnus, stated, "If God had not given us a vessel, His other gifts would have been to no avail." Without the vessel, the work cannot proceed. But what is this vessel and what does it offer to us in terms of soul work?

To the alchemist, the vessel was a literal container, usually made of glass, within which the physical operations of transmutation took place. It was in the vessel that the base materials were placed. They were then subjected to heat and various modes of change, moving them toward the goal of the *stone* or *lapis*, often referred to as *gold*. In order to aid these processes of transformation, the alchemists would subject the material to various operations such as *separatio*, *calcinatio*, *mortificatio*, and *coagulatio*, among many others. Each operation intended to hasten the work of nature, which the alchemists said was the movement from base metal to the *philosopher's stone*. In psychological language, it is the work of redeeming the complex in service of the soul. James Hillman says it this way:

> The alchemists had an excellent image for the transformation of suffering and symptom into a value of soul. A goal of the alchemical process was the pearl of great price. The pearl starts off as a bit of grit, a neurotic symptom or complaint, a bothersome irritant in one's secret inside flesh, which no defensive shell can protect oneself from. This is coated over, worked at day in and day out, until the

grit one day is a pearl; yet it still must be fished up from the depths and pried loose. Then when the grit is redeemed, it is worn. It must be worn on the warm skin to keep its luster: the redeemed complex which once caused suffering is exposed to public view as a virtue. The esoteric treasure gained through occult work becomes an exoteric splendor. To get rid of the symptom means to get rid of the chance to gain what may one day be of greatest value, even if at first an unbearable irritant, lowly and disguised.[25]

All of this happens in the vessel. The vessel, however, must be carefully tended. There are frequent warnings in many alchemical texts about the need to pay rigorous attention to the condition of the vessel in order to assure the success of the effort. In particular, they were concerned about the ability of the vessel to tolerate the effects generated by the various operations—pressure, heat, rising vapors—so as to not spoil the work through a failure of the vessel.

The seventeenth-century alchemist Philalethes wrote,

> Let your glass distilling vessel be round or oval. . . . Let the height of the vessel's neck be about one palm, hand-breadth, and let the glass be clear and thick (the thicker the better, so long as it is clear and clean, and permits you to distinguish what is going on within). . . . The glass should be strong in order to prevent the vapours which arise from our embryo bursting the vessel. Let the mouth of the vessel be *very* carefully and effectively secured by means of a thick layer of sealing wax.[26]

His guidelines suggest much for our work with soul. First, we are told that we must attain some clarity in order to note "what is going on within." We must be able to see through our projections and defenses, our strategies and fictions, in hopes of seeing things as they are. No small feat! A degree of courage is in order here, asking us to look into our psychic lives with a clear and discerning eye.

Secondly, we are instructed that the work requires a degree of strength; that the "glass should be strong" so that in the course of our efforts, it does not break. We all have known times when we were broken by the events in our lives. We felt shattered and fragile, the vessel compromised. It takes strength to engage the energies emerging from the psyche. It takes a strong vessel to engage the wild images, surges of grief and remorse, the difficult memories that return, the agitations and depressions, desires, and longings. The vessel, strengthened by our attention and devotion, becomes capable, over time, of containing it all. In fact, that is one of the central goals of the work. It is not about resolving our issues or repairing the past but becoming more spacious and capable of holding all that psyche and life bring to us. Again, not an easy achievement.

The poet Federico García Lorca declared that our ability to engage in this work requires *disciplina y pasión*, discipline and passion to move the work forward. Discipline is the effort and muscle of vesseling, without which the vessel breaks. We all want to invoke the wild, passionate, creative energies in our lives, but without discipline, without containment, we will burn out. We only need to think of many of the ones we have lost over the years—Monroe, Joplin, Holiday, Hendrix, Morrison, Cobain—burning brilliantly but without sufficient containment, reduced to ash. Part of the strength we require to do the work of cultivating soul is relational. We cannot do this work in isolation. As Jung noted, "The soul cannot exist without its other side, which is always found in a 'You.'"[27]

And lastly, we can hear in Philalethes's words the dictum, "Let the mouth of the vessel be *very* carefully and effectively secured." This is the essential practice of restraint, one that we often struggle to follow. In *Psychology and Alchemy*, Jung writes,

"The *vas bene clausum* (well-sealed vessel) is a precautionary measure very frequently mentioned in alchemy . . . the idea is to protect what is within from the intrusion and admixture of what is without, as well as to prevent it from escaping."[28] What is cooking in the vessel must not be allowed to escape or leak, nor is it good to add to the material once the work has been engaged. If this occurs, we run the risk of diluting the work or spoiling it entirely. We often share an insight too soon or expose a newly inspired project to others prematurely, and suddenly the idea fades and the insight withers. Learning to seal the mouth and "treat the work-in-progress as a secret" is a vital necessity in the work. Let it simmer, ripen, and mature. Let the material become what it desires to become, not for our sake but for the sake of soul.

Vessels separate as well as contain, offering us a way to identify the particular piece that is presenting itself and calling for our attention. In a very real way, we cannot cultivate a psychological or soulful life without containment. Hillman, once again, reminds us that "psyche appears to be only what it contains."[29] In other words, without our capacity to notice and attend, reflect, witness, engage, and love, we would be bereft of any psychic life. When we practice these *arts of vesseling*, we extend an intimacy to what is moving in the soul. This happens through the slow, continuous building of the vessel. Think of therapy, for example, and the ongoing repetition, hour upon hour, turning over the materials of psyche—images, dreams, moods, memories, fantasies, confusions, complexes, relationships—all requiring a space to be witnessed and deepened, allowing the *masa confusa* to slowly yield some new precious drop of insight.

The image of the vessel is ancient and was most notably developed in the work of alchemy. Carl Jung reclaimed alchemy from obscurity when he discovered, hidden within the arcane imagery of the alchemists, a profound description of the processes of psyche. He recovered a stunning array of images, metaphors, and operations that offer us a way of approaching the work of soul that is immediate and tangible rather than abstract and conceptual. Images of kings and queens, fountains and snakes, peacocks and ravens, dragons and furnaces, filled the depictions of alchemical texts. They worked with the materials of the physical world—lead, iron, sulfur, mercury, salt—all inferring an interior resonance with the ways of psyche. We have all felt leaden from time to time: slow, heavy, weighed down by life. And we have all tasted the bitterness of regret, the raw salt mines of our wounds that we return to over and over again and bathe with our salty tears. The rich metaphors offered by alchemy lend themselves to a more imaginative psychology, one alive with soul.

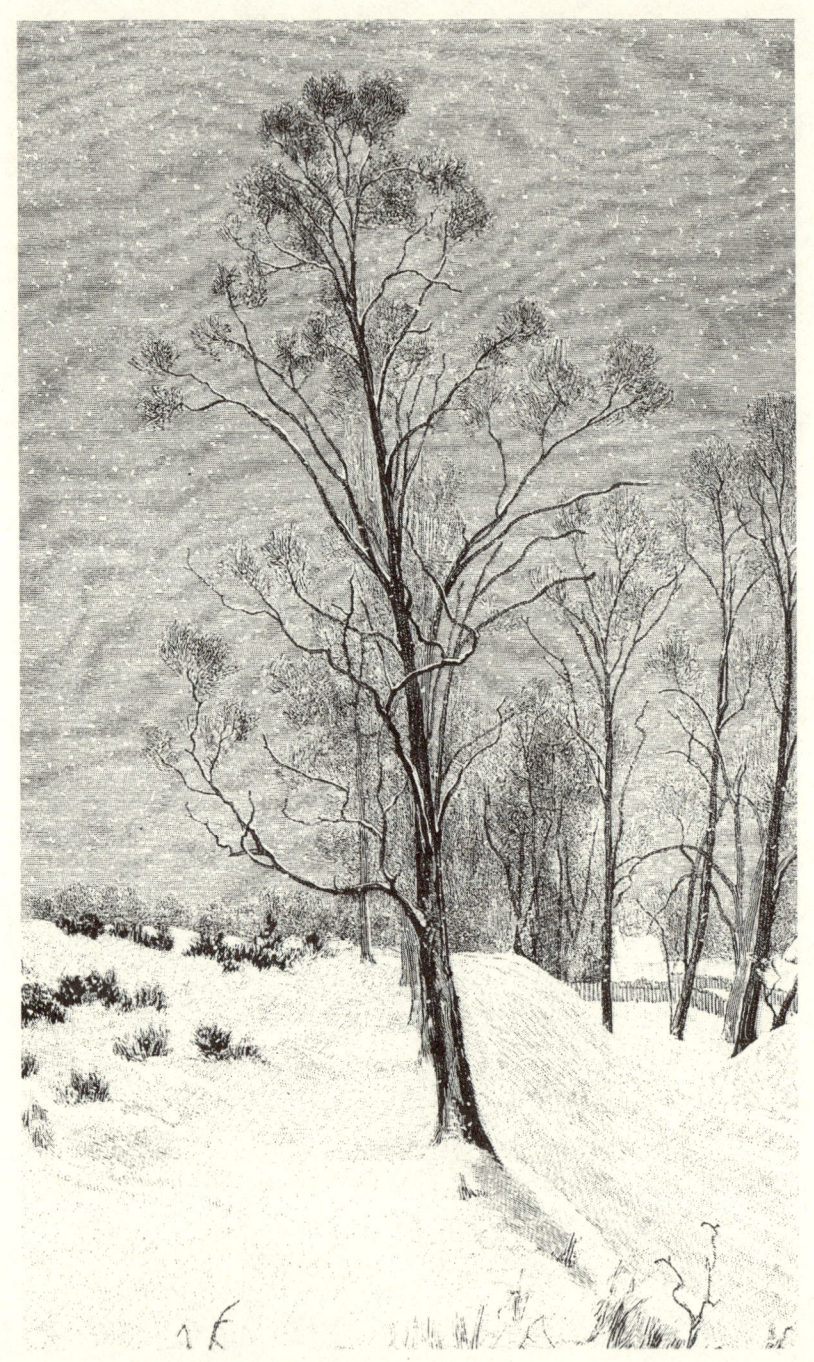

Nine

The Gift of Restraint

IN A SERIES OF TALKS I offered in early 2018, called *Living a Soulful Life and Why It Matters*, I shared multiple ways to see the daily manifestations of soul, how it reveals itself through our encounters with wounds, images, creativity, friendship, grief, the ancestors, and more. Underlying these epiphanic displays are the *values* that soul holds, values that were shaped over thousands of years and that emerged as central to our survival as a species. In these times of disorientation and uncertainty, recovering these essential nodes of being may help us navigate the coming challenges in a more considered way.

We begin our exploration of the values of soul in an unexpected territory: *restraint*. The choice is intentional. In an age of instant gratification and excessive consumption, the value of restraint must come acutely into view. We are drowning in our possessions and our garbage. We are exhausting the very fabric of the world, consuming the equivalent of 1.5 Earths every year. Astonishingly, if everyone on the planet lived like members of the United States, we would need 4.9 Earths per year to meet the demand. The depletion process is far outstripping the regeneration capacities of the planet. Restraint, however, is one of the least developed spiritual values we have. It may not be as sexy as courage and boldness. Nor is it the most popular at the party. Exuberance and abundance get that award. Restraint is more introspective, contained, and held back. It is a bit austere, preferring not doing to doing.

There are both internal and external forms of restraint.

Internally, restraint invites a pause, a breath, a moment of reflection. How rarely we do this—pause, breathe, reflect. It is a core practice in the art of ripening. We must grant time and space for things to ripen and mature. Insights, intuitions, encounters, and dreams, all require time to incubate and consolidate into something substantial. We continually reveal and share things too soon, rarely allowing a new revelation time to mature and become part of our psychic ground. We need to hold, contain, and cook the material before sharing it with the world. It must be allowed to go through its own process of distillation prior to being revealed to questioning eyes. The value of restraint acknowledges this truth and creates a space where something can take shape according to its nature.

Our constant management and manipulation of all things psychic reveal a lack of faith in the movements of soul. It is essential to practice noninterference, letting the deep work of soul go on without our interventions. We must, as Jung says (quoting the great German mystic Meister Eckhart), "let go of ourselves."[30] And, as Jung notes, this is an "art" that "opens the door to the way." Or as Jung said, paraphrasing Eckhart, "We must let go and let be." Restraint is a form of trust in the deep workings of soul.

When we honor the value of restraint, the door to genuine receiving opens. Grasping to satisfy every hunger leaves no room for the generosity of the world to find us. Restraint is a form of faithfulness: faith that we will be cared for; that we will be offered kindness and care from others when our hearts and souls are troubled. Restraint opens the aperture where we can be found.

There is a marvelous tempering of psyche by the heat generated through nonaction. It is a *via negativa*, a path of negation. To restrain means "to bind back" and "to hold back." This creates heat through the tension of resistance. It is this heat that creates contour and shape in our interior lives. You can feel it when you hesitate to act on some impulse, desire, or craving. Space is created when we let go of something. It requires strength and fortitude, commitment, and devotion. It is a move toward holding steady, allowing the deeper and often hidden rhythms of soul to emerge.

The lyrical poet of *duende*, Federico García Lorca, called us to live in the dynamic tension between discipline and passion. Restraint is a form of discipline. It offers a holding space, a vessel, in the old alchemical language, for cooking the raw material, the *prima materia*, into a new shape.

We place a great deal of emphasis on desire, longing, expression, and wildness in our lives. All of this is beautiful and necessary. Without its other side, however, we lack the tempering that is provided through the tension of restraint. It is possible that holding back is as necessary as action is to the soul.

Restraint offers a powerful antidote to our self-focused psychologies and our consumptive economics. It loosens the tight grip of the self as the sole signifier of importance. Through the agency of restraint, we can address the needs and voices of others, human and more-than-human, in our concerns. Many traditions practiced gestures of restraint, such as fasting, as a means of returning the individual, repeatedly, back to the ground of humility.

Externally, at the heart of restraint is an awareness that our well-being is entangled with the well-being of all others. Many myths and fairy tales speak of the necessity of restraint, particularly in terms of our relations with our plant and animal kin. These wisdom tales warn of the dangers that accompany selfishness, greed, and taking more than necessary. To practice self-control is to maintain the tender equilibrium between the worlds. In many of these tales, the animals would withdraw their consent to be offered to the human world when we acted out of balance. Consequently, the game disappeared, and the people suffered. The intuitive knowledge of the people was meant to prevent wholesale depletion of what it was they required to survive. We have forgotten this life-preserving value in our times. Overfishing, mountaintop removal, clear-cutting of forests, loss of topsoil, emptying and poisoning of aquifers are all outgrowths of the failure to practice restraint.

Restraint moves contrary to the goals of acquisition and accumulation. It is, rather, a value that serves the commons, arising as it does from our long story of mutual survival. It is rooted in an embedded truth that we have endured together. Our survival is possible only in collaboration with the many others with whom we share this stunning world.

The Iroquois Confederacy in the Northeast territory of the continent practiced a principle of considering the seventh generation in their deliberations. Any action they took would have to be sustainable for those generations yet to come. This is the embodiment of cultural restraint.

There is a potent connection between restraint and humility. The action/nonaction of restraint suggests that there is a value in holding back and limiting the movements we are wanting to make. Restraint recognizes the dangers of continuous growth, addition, and consumption. It leans into the wisdom of moderation— another word not praised in our *no-limits* culture. In an age of "You can have it all," there is an implicit entitlement to consume, extract, and possess. What drives this rapacious appetite is an interior sense of emptiness and lack. We have forgotten the *primary satisfactions*[31] in our lives and have been left with a deep absence in our core.

Restraint, along with patience, offers a pause, a moment of reflection when we can take in the needs of another. In the space of holding back, we recognize that our well-being is intricately entwined with the health of the commons. To act in a selfish manner is to put our own lives in jeopardy. To take too much disturbs the delicate balance of watersheds and communities. Restraint asks us to cherish the fact of our mutually entangled lives. We are inseparable from all that surrounds us.

In the coming years, we will inevitably be required to reduce not only our consumption but also our sense of needing so much to live a rich and soulful life. Let us come to see the value of restraint, of creating space through the practice of not doing. It may be there that we find ourselves escorted into the chamber of what it is the soul truly longs for.

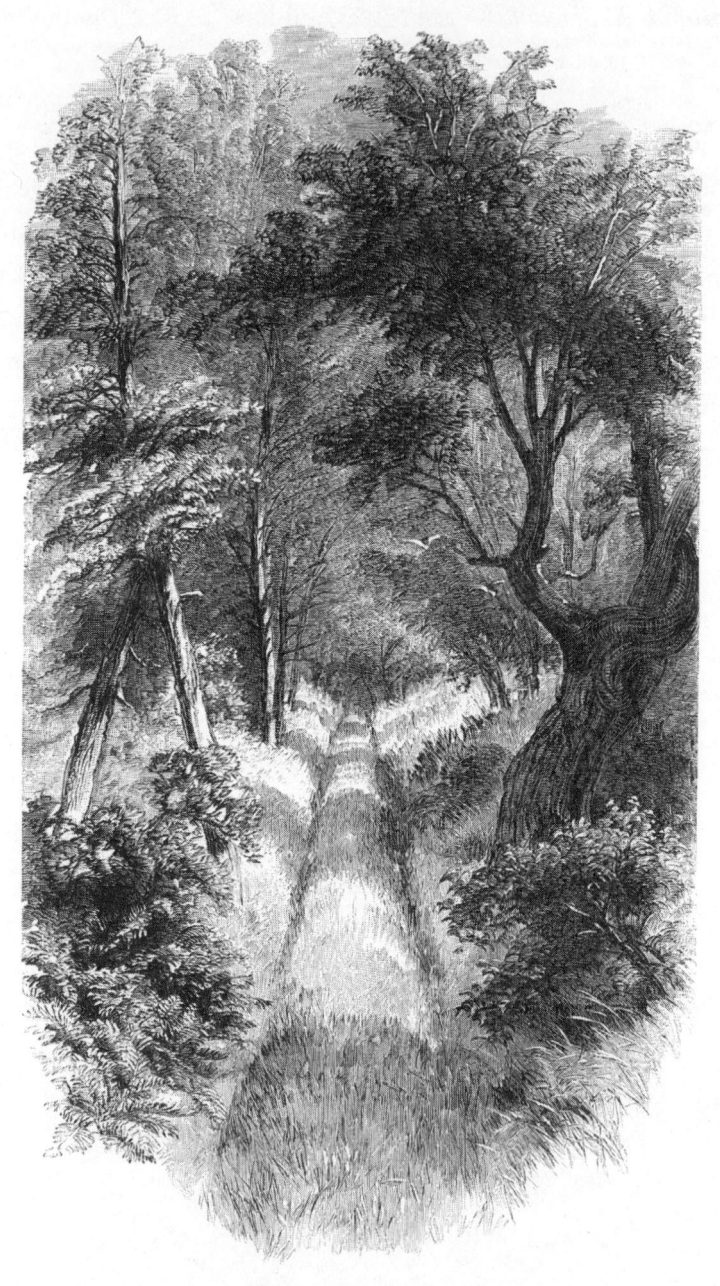

Ten

The Value of Repetition

OUR EXPLORATION OF SOUL VALUES began with the often-neglected practice of restraint. We now venture into another underappreciated quality of soul, and that is repetition. Like restraint, repetition is not glamorous or sexy. It is ordinary and ebbs and flows through our daily lives in both conscious and unconscious ways.

In this culture, we struggle with the idea of repetition, anything that seems too familiar. We want things to be novel, new and improved, the latest. There is nothing wrong with this. It does, however, tinge the old and traditional with a feeling of being antiquated and outdated. (It is interesting to note that for many traditional people, anything new was approached with an attitude of suspicion. Where did this come from? Will it serve the people? How will it affect the land?)

We live in a society that prizes constant innovation and novelty. The singular focus on growth and development has provided us with many new devices and technologies and granted us a degree of ease seldom known by our ancestors. It also casts a long and weighty shadow. Embedded in this ideology is an obsession with progress.

Progress is holy scripture in this culture. It is the one-directional arrow of time and productivity that surrounds us and informs us daily. We feel the constant pressure to have more, be more, and achieve more. There is something inherent in the concept of progress, however, that leaves a residue of discontent in its wake. The better life is always just beyond the horizon, awaiting the arrival of the latest product, accomplishment, or discovery. We are taught to crave what is next, the up-and-coming. The old and familiar are considered outworn and outdated. We are quick to discard anything considered old—including people—leaving us skimming the surface, carried along on the swift-moving current of progress.

This pressure is felt in our psychological lives as well. There is an ongoing focus on improving and being better. How we are is rarely good enough. We must constantly strive to grow. Growth and progress are the two primary imperatives within psychology. Consequently, discontent is built into the way we approach our psychological lives. The focus settles on what we do not have, what we have not achieved, and the progress we have not made.

Soul, on the other hand, values repetition. Repetition is a form of sustained attention, returning us repeatedly to a place, a person, or a practice, which engenders depth and familiarity. It is in the very essence of repetition that we come to know something more intimately, whether a partner, a friend, or our own interior worlds. Any movement toward depth requires repeated contact. Gary Snyder, the Zen poet and nature philosopher, wrote that "getting intimate with nature and our own wild natures is a matter of going face to face many times."[32] There is no depth without excavating and digging into the marrow of what matters to soul and culture. Repetition is a form of courtship.

Soul engages repetition in many ways. Consider how often we are brought back to the cave of our wounds. We are taken to these places, often unwillingly, as a way of remaining close by, not straying too far from something essential in the making of soul.

It is through the ongoing entanglement with our suffering that flavor and shape are delivered into our lives. James Hillman says our wounds and traumas are "salt mines from which we gain a precious essence and without which the soul cannot live."[33]

Our sense of discontent, in part, arises out of neglecting the core practices that were repeated and unbroken for hundreds of generations. Now, under the fevered pitch of individualism and the heroic ego, the original practices that wove the individual and the community together have been largely forgotten. Consequently, the ritual of life is reduced to the routine of existence. That is repetition without soul. That is the drone of addiction. That is repetition that deadens.

Soulful repetition offers a way to foster the art of remembering. We live in a culture that encourages amnesia and anesthesia; we forget, and we go numb. In our obsession with progress, the roots of memory have deteriorated and faded. "Repetition," says anthropologist Elizabeth Marshall Thomas, "is a form of permanence."[34] This was vital for our survival. The dances, rituals, songs, and stories, the intricate knowledge of plants and animals, how to shape adult human beings, all combined to form a means of maintaining the trail through the world. The continuity of wisdom passed on from generation to generation was crucial to our ongoing survival. When we forget the old ways of our ancestors, we lose contact with the roots of wisdom.

We live in an ongoing tension between forgetting and remembering. Nearly all enduring cultures developed practices designed to help us remember three central things: who we are, where we belong, and what is sacred. Prayer, meditation, and ritual are, at root, designed to help us stay awake. These practices serve to sustain the ground of remembrance, which is, in turn, a form of permanence.

Soul exerts its gravitational pull repeatedly in our lifetime, calling us into the rich loam of image, emotion, memory, dream, and longing. Living cultures exert a similar compelling quality, drawing the community together through the repetitive gestures of ritual, initiatory cycles, pilgrimages to sacred places, and the ongoing rounds of tending the village. Oral traditions are rooted in the rhythms of repetition. The great stories were told over and over again. It was in the retelling that the multiple layers hidden in the tale were slowly revealed. Our earliest shared acts were designed to weave and knit the community together, and then by extension, into the surrounding field of nature and cosmos. Repetition serves to continuously renew and reaffirm the entangled nature of our beings.

Soulful repetition is not boring or bland. It is musical, rhythmic, and enduring. We require touchstones of return to stay connected to what matters to soul and culture. Repetition is a gesture of affection, of fidelity. We return again and again to tend what it is we love and, by so doing, we keep it alive and vital.

REFLECTION QUESTION: In what ways do you nourish the ritual of everyday life? What core practices help sustain your intimacy with soul?

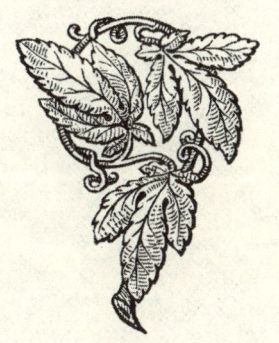

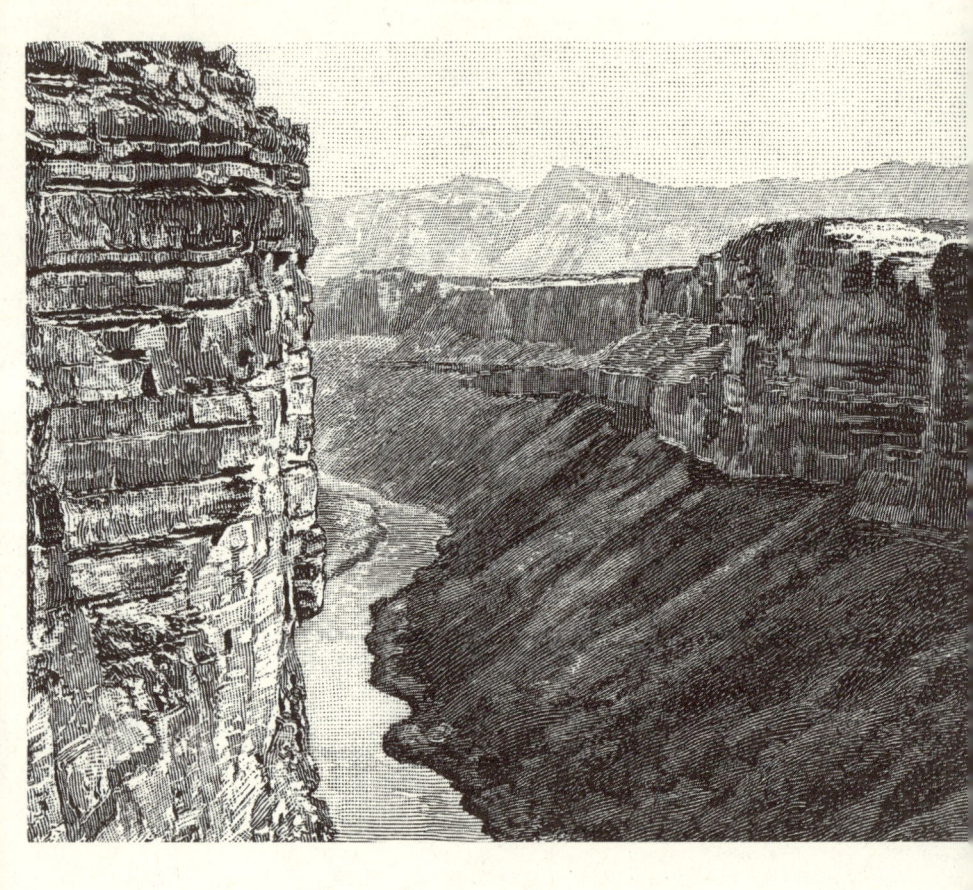

Eleven

Approaching Geologic Speed

MOST EVERY DAY IN MY WORK, I hear how rushed people feel in their day-to-day lives. I feel the same pressure to keep things moving. There is always more to do, another deadline to meet. We are moving at a breathless pace much of the time, and in some way, we have come to see this as normal. We live in a cult of terminal velocity, a type of mania that consumes us with constant motion. Much is lost in this frenzied fidelity to speed.

Consider this: The May/June 2015 edition of *Orion* magazine included an excerpt from Robert Macfarlane's new book, *Landmarks*. In this short piece, Macfarlane shares his love of language, especially words that speak of our relationship with the living landscape. He had been collecting place-words for more than a decade and he shared some of his discoveries. A few of my favorites include *ammil*, "a Devon term meaning 'the sparkle of morning sunlight through hoar-frost'"; *blinter*, "a northern Scots word meaning 'a cold dazzle,' connoting especially 'the radiance of winter stars on a clear night'"; and *pirr*, "meaning 'a light breath of wind, such as will make a cat's paw on the water.'"[35]

These words kindle a feeling of intimacy with the land and cosmos. What struck me in his article—in addition to the wonderful inclusion of these words—was his reporting that in 2007, the *Oxford Junior Dictionary* decided to omit a swath of words from its latest edition, deeming these words irrelevant to the minds of children. The list was chilling: *acorn, adder, ash, beech, bluebell, buttercup, catkin, dandelion, fern, heather, heron, ivy, king-fisher, lark, mistletoe, nectar, newt, otter, pasture,* and *willow.* As if to say, these words were no longer a part of the world in which children lived. In their place, the dictionary included *attachment, blog, broadband, bullet-point, celebrity, chatroom, MP3 player,* and *voice-mail.*

There is no arguing that the new words are reflective of the enveloping world of today's youth, revealing the much greater emphasis on the technological and virtual over the natural and sensual. This change, however, reflects a diminishment in our imaginations, in the very way we touch the world. It is a loss of the intimacy, based on close observation and prolonged attention, that appreciates the particulars of a place or a person. This kind of connection takes time, slowing downward and entering into a reciprocal rhythm. The new words that were added to the dictionary reflect an attitude altogether based on speed. And this was ten years ago. I can only imagine what further winnowing has occurred in the language that previously escorted us into the actual, breathing world.

I share this with you as a way of calling attention to a fundamental disorder of our time: *speed.* We are addicted to speed, with the demand for faster internet and cell phones, clipped conversations via text and email, fast food, and virtual friendships. There is a gnawing feeling that we will never catch up with the demands of our lives.

Speed can rob us of the moment, and can so thin the exchange between our body and the other—whether oak, friend, or beloved cat—that we fail to take in the fragrance of the exchange. In these times, we are marooned in our own vacant interiority, spinning and twisting, lacking the touch that affirms contact. We are dying a bit every day from this lack of connection.

I remember listening to Brother David Steindl-Rast, a Benedictine monk, give a talk many years ago in Marin County, California. I do not remember the overall theme of his talk, but as is often the case with Brother David, it circulated around the heart. At one point in his talk, he shared that the Chinese spell the word "busy" with two ideograms that mean "heart" and "killing." We all gasped as he shared this idea. We pride ourselves on how busy we are as if to suggest worth and value are attained by our exhaustion. And yet, our obsession with speed increases daily.

What does our heart require in order to feel alive and connected to the wider expanse of swifts and swallowtails, lichen, and Mozart? One essential thing we need is time. We need to slow down and come into the spaciousness of not doing. This is such an un-American thought, but I know it to be true.

Many years ago, I spent some time in West Africa, visiting my friend Malidoma Somé in the village of Dano. The first three days after I arrived in Dano were somewhat torturous. The heat was oppressive. We spent hours sitting as the elders chatted or sat in silence. We would move on occasion to stay sheltered by the shade. I struggled with the level of inaction, wondering internally when we were going to *do* something. What I noticed over time, however, was how busy I was in my mind, in my habitual pattern of activity. I slowly began to relax and come back into a rhythm I now know is indigenous to the soul. I began to value this time of stillness, as I recalled the old rhythms of soul.

One of my most memorable teachings about slowing down came from my mentor Clarke Berry, a Jungian analyst with whom I apprenticed following licensure. I was young and I knew I needed a mentor, someone who could teach me the art of sitting with others in therapy. The Jung Institute in San Francisco referred me to Clarke along with other analysts, but when I met him I knew I was in the right place. Our first meeting more than four decades ago was unforgettable. We sat down and Clarke reached over to his left, placed his hand on a large rock lying on a table, and said, "This is my clock. I operate at geologic speed. And if you are going to work with the soul, you need to learn this rhythm because this is how the soul moves." Then he pointed to a small clock also sitting there and added, "It hates this." What an amazing thing to tell this young therapist. It is the single most important thing I ever learned about therapy, about working with the soul.

In those moments when we are able to experience the rhythm of the soul, we are opened to an *ordinary mysticism* that reveals the grandeur of what surrounds us. We find ourselves living in a sacred cosmos, flourishing with beauty and potency. Only a people unable to apprehend this majesty could treat the earth with such violence. Speed blinds us to this splendor, diminishes our vision, and narrows the aperture of the heart.

James Cowan, in his magical book *Letters from a Wild State*, says,

> We have allowed the language of materialism to drown out the last echo of the inner chorus we once knew by heart. The song denoting our primal concerns has been submerged under the wash of blasphemies that masquerade as our reason for existence. We have allowed ourselves to become lifelong victims of an economic rather than a spiritual process. In so doing, we've adopted the illusion that the raucous sounds of satiety are an acceptable substitute for the music of the spheres.[36]

Geologic speed—the rhythm of eons, of millennia—is etched deep in our bones. When we grant ourselves the time and pace of stone, we come into a deep memory of who we are, where we belong, and what is sacred. We remember the values associated with this ancient cadence, among them patience, restraint, and reciprocity.

Patience helps us to recognize that we live in a multicentric cosmos where everything possesses its own interiority, its own shimmering essence. Patience enables us to witness and listen, to welcome and honor the dignity that is inherent in all things. Whereas we are conditioned to push things along and make things happen, patience enables us to allow things to ripen and season, itself a word that invites slow time into our imagination. We must simply wait for the season when the apple is ready to ripen.

Restraint, as I have alluded to, is akin to a slow inbreath that can help place ourselves back into the eternal conversation between self and world. It takes time to have a conversation of depth, to create a space of invitation and intimacy. Restraint carves fertile openings in the spaces between our interior lives and the surrounding field of the animate earth. Here, in the space of holding and pausing, we come into the grace of slowness, the pace of stone.

Reciprocity is the embodiment of the fact that we come alive because of this entanglement. We live in a dynamic system of give-and-take. This is an ancient knowing, reflected in the many rituals of gratitude that traditional people celebrate knowing that we live in a gifting cosmos. Remembering to offer a simple gesture of thankfulness places us back into the conversation with the living world.

Some time ago, my son and I took a road trip to the Southwest. We visited several sites that carry the pace of stone. As we walked through the ancient pueblos of Mesa Verde and Chaco Canyon, I could hear the voices of the ancestors singing and talking. While at Mesa Verde, I had the opportunity to enter one of the kivas, underground spaces often dedicated to ritual. In this space, I encountered a silence that deeply affected me. My mind went quiet, and I felt connected to the unbroken arc of time. I encountered a similar silence in the grand plaza at Chaco Canyon. It was a silence that enveloped everything. My son reminded me, however, that during its height, the plaza was filled with the sounds of the village: drums; rituals; markets brimming with people, daily gossip, and the murmur of children.

We stopped at one particularly enchanted place called Rock Art Canyon in Arizona. The canyon is nestled between sheer rock walls with a year-round stream flowing through it. Etched into the walls were hundreds of petroglyphs, some dating back nine thousand years. Images of elk, bighorn sheep, shamans, and stars, beautiful geometric patterns, and antlered figures. The images were mesmerizing, and I was transported to another time, one rich with shades of a vibrant village, and a pervasive sense of the sacred. The images carried a numinous character that pulled me into another world. For many hours, my son and I had the canyon to ourselves. For a brief time, I was able to meet these ancient others with my own pace of stone. As evening approached, we reluctantly took our leave.

Geologic speed weaves through our minds, bodies, and souls, shaping our instincts, dreams, and longings. In our modern frenzied culture, however, with its twin obsessions of progress and speed, we rarely address this intrinsic mode of being. We are more familiar with the din of the machine, and the hum of the computer, but rarely the songs of the soul. What matters most to our soul is found in places of slowness, the terrain of geologic speed. For the sake of our souls and the soul of the world, slow down and come into the rich loam of the waiting world.

Soul Work

Take an afternoon and sit on your porch, in a park, near a river-bank, and DO NOTHING. Notice the thoughts and feelings that arise. Later, when you have time, write about what you experienced. Be welcoming of all that arises, even the difficult and uncomfortable things.

Be as mindful as you can of the pace you inhabit in any given day. Notice if the rhythm is compulsively busy. And then try to notice what happens when you slow down and enter the stream of connection with the daylight, the wind, the sounds of the city, birdsong, cricket, or silence.

Take time in the evening to allow the light to fade, then enter the darkness and sense this ancient mode of perception. Behind the well-lit areas of our modern minds lies the ancient soul, and it is here that we most readily recall geologic speed. Later, take some time and reflect on your experience in the night, or share your discoveries with a friend or your partner. Invite them to join you in the stillness.

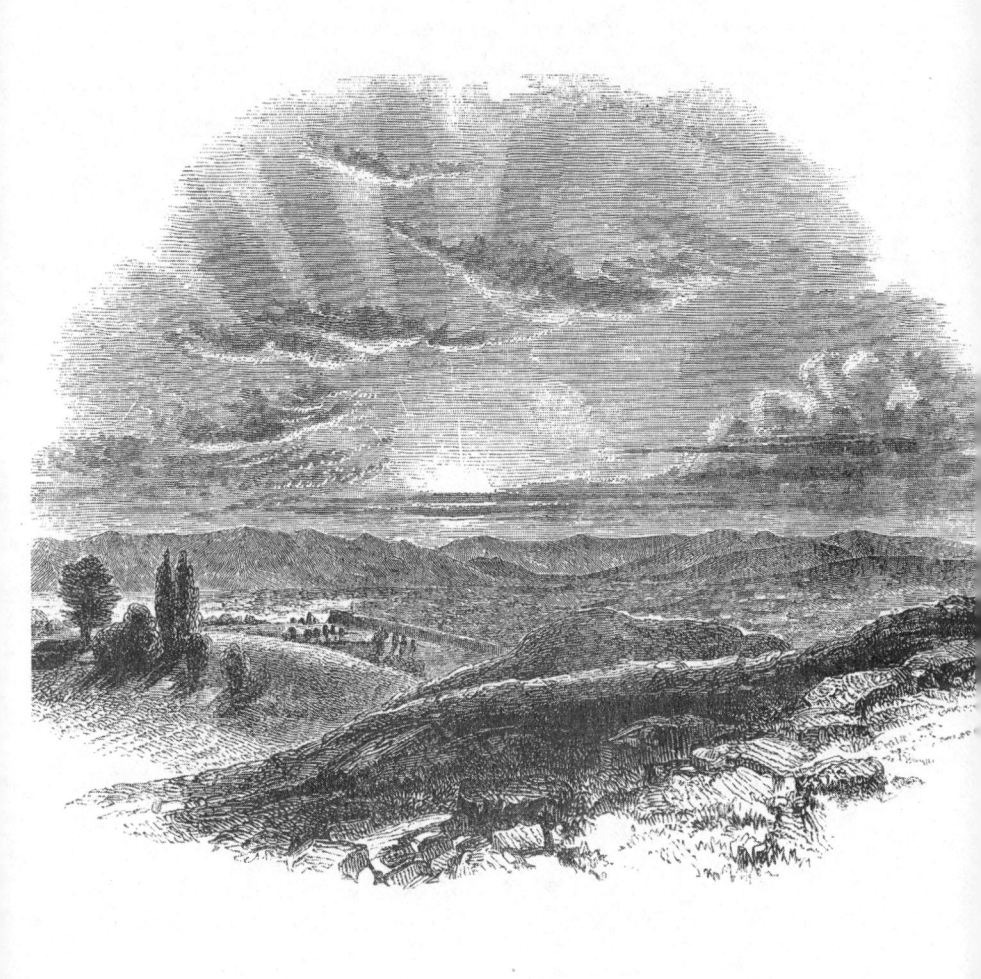

Twelve

The Generous Heart
The Gift of Self-Compassion

You can search throughout the entire universe for someone
who is more deserving of your love and affection than you
are yourself, and that person is not to be found anywhere.
You, yourself, as much as anybody in the entire
universe, deserve your love and affection.[37]
—BUDDHA

AT THE HEART OF EVERY SPIRITUAL TRADITION, we find the
teaching of compassion. Through the gate of compassion, we are
invited to enter the wider conversation with all life. Compassion
binds us with all things through the shared encounter with suffering. The word "compassion" comes from the Latin *com pati*,
"to suffer with." It is through our shared experience with loss,
sorrow, and pain that we deepen our connection with one another
and enter the commons of the soul.

But how are we with *self-compassion*? Too often our caring
is reserved for those outside of ourselves, as though we have not
earned the right to kindness. We struggle with judgments and
resist offering gestures of mercy to ourselves. Yet, every one of us
knows loss and defeat, loneliness, and failure. We hurt and harm
others, are hurt and harmed by others; we close our hearts to the
world and often choose self-protection as a way of life.

Bringing compassion to our suffering is an act of generosity. It helps us remember that we, too, are part of this breathing, pulsing world and worthy of compassion. We are reminded that, by the mere fact of our being here, we qualify for the soothing waters of compassion. We can then come out of our sheltered world of self-scrutiny and make our way back into the fuller embrace of our belonging.

When I work with groups on the topic of self-compassion, I often begin by describing our time together as a project in "non-self-improvement." So often, our efforts at change in our lives mask subtle and not-so-subtle acts of self-hatred. We attack portions of our life with a vengeance, fully believing that our weakness or inadequacy, our neediness, or our failures are the reasons for our suffering and *if only* we could be free of them, then we would enter into a state of perfection; all would be well. Our obsession with perfection is itself a strategy that we cling to, to overcome our feelings of being outside the wall of welcome.

Giving up our muscular agendas of self-improvement is an act of kindness. It says that by befriending our life, we deepen our capacity to welcome what is, what comes, and whoever arrives at the interior door of our soul's house. We do not often get to decide who or what shows up in the "guest house,"[38] as Rumi says, but we can cultivate an atmosphere of curiosity and receptivity. Self-compassion gradually becomes one of the basic elements of maturation. We slowly relinquish the harsh program of ridding ourselves of our outcast brothers and sisters for the sake of fitting in; we simply set another place at the table.

This is not to say that we do not seek change. At a recent gathering, a man said to me, "I noticed that you don't talk about progress in your work." I said, "No. I don't see the soul moving in a linear way, from Point A to Point B. Sometimes it moves downward or sideways, sometimes it regresses, and at other times it holds still and does not move. Progress is one of our culture's most cherished fictions, but it can do great harm when applied to the life of the soul. As soon as we are not moving forward or progressing, we feel something is wrong and that we are failing, so we redouble our efforts. What self-compassion offers us is the space and breath to listen and take notice of how our soul is moving at this moment; what it is asking us to pay attention to at this time."

He then asked if I was okay with having goals. I said, "Well, I'm not real comfortable with goals either, but if I had to use that language, I would say that the goal of this work is to extend the level of participation of the soul as widely and deeply as possible. One of the deepest sources of depression for the soul is a diminished range of participation in our life. To be fully alive: that would be the goal." This is the change we truly long for.

The foundations of self-compassion arise from the fertile ground of belonging. Belonging confers a feeling of worth and value, which in turn filters into our whole being like a blessing. This gently translates into a relationship with oneself that is respectful and caring. Herein lies our problem: For many of us, the experience of belonging has been fractured and frustrated. We often feel as though we are living outside the warmth of a recognizable welcome. In this state of exile and loneliness, we feel unworthy of compassion or kindness. I have heard countless times in my practice someone saying, "I feel unlovable." It is particularly challenging to cultivate a feeling of compassion for oneself in an atmosphere of self-judgment and hatred.

Nearly everywhere I go to teach, there is an ongoing call for some dressing to heal the wounds around belonging. Fortunately, almost every one of us has been able to forge some friendships, small circles of welcome, even if we feel they are provisional. This can be enough to help stimulate the practice of self-compassion. One of the working definitions that I am playing with is that self-compassion is the "internalized village." Pause for a moment and think about how we tend to respond to a friend who is suffering. Usually, we feel an immediate opening in our hearts of caring and sympathy toward their pain. We do not typically recoil in judgment or condemnation and yet, that is often how we respond to our own moments of pain. Imagine, instead, that these dear people in our lives are dwelling inside of us, that the little village in our world has been taken into our hearts. Now, when suffering arises, our interior friend can say to us, "Be gentle. Be kind. Be compassionate with this suffering part of your life." It is soothing to imagine the village residing inside our chest. Perhaps the Golden Rule needs an addendum: "Do unto yourself as you would do unto others." This *pilgrimage of friendship* toward our own life is essential to any move we wish to make into the larger and more fulfilling life that awaits us.

Self-compassion is a fierce and challenging practice. Every day we are asked to sit with pieces of our interior world that lie outside of what we find acceptable and welcome. We must explore our *learned responses* to our places of suffering and actively engage these pieces of soul life. We have often treated these parts of ourselves with indifference, if not outright contempt. I recently invited a group of men to share in a ritual where we turned toward these outcast parts of our lives with compassion and apology. The ritual was deceptively simple. We placed five large stones on the ground near the base of an immense ancient oak. As I drummed and we all sang, men approached the stones, knelt on the ground, and each man slowly lifted one stone off the ground. In their minds and imaginations, they were seeing an outcast brother lying under the stone. He had been weighed down under it and unable to stand upright again until this gesture of kindness was offered. Men wept as they lifted the stone off these parts of themselves and slowly welcomed the fragments of life these brothers carried for them. It was beautiful and healing.

Lifting the stones off the backs of these parts of our lives may help to restore what poet David Whyte calls a state of innocence. I cautiously use this term as well, not to insinuate some child-like state of purity, but to suggest that through self-compassion, we are offered the possibility of new beginnings. No part of us releases in a state of judgment. The overly critical mind creates a state of contraction, whereas compassion softens and makes possible a state of beginning, a fresh and unshaped ripeness. Rebecca del Rio offers this poem as an invitation to renewal and beginnings:

Prescription for the Disillusioned

Come new to this day.
Remove the rigid
overcoat of experience,
the notion of knowing,
the beliefs that cloud
your vision.

Leave behind the stories
of your life. Spit out the
sour taste of unmet expectation.
Let the stale scent of what-ifs
waft back into the swamp
of your useless fears.

Arrive curious, without the armor
of certainty, the plans and planned
results of the life you've imagined.
Live the life that chooses you, new
every breath, every blink of
your astonished eyes.[39]

Self-compassion is not an event but an ongoing daily practice. It is *the* root practice for our inner life and for our relational lives. I remember giving many talks on shame and sharing how we want to be in loving relationships while simultaneously hating ourselves. Our ability to receive love is proportional to our capacity to welcome all of who we are. Self-compassion is a skill that needs to be exercised and developed regularly for us to remain open and available to life. It is the gift of a generous heart.

PART III

Meanwhile, the World Goes On

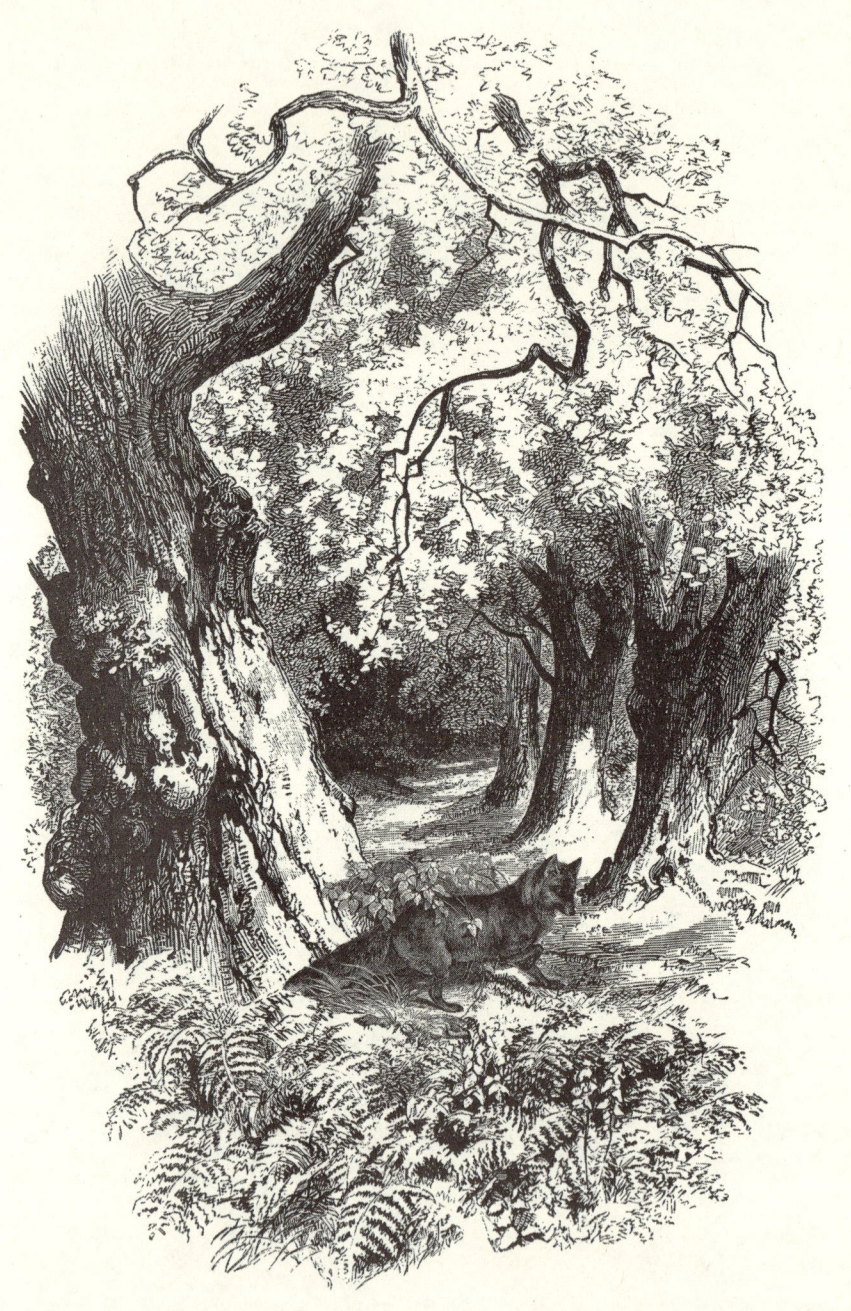

Thirteen

A Beautiful and Strange Otherness

I WAS RECENTLY in the pine forests of Northern Minnesota to teach at the Minnesota Men's Conference. I was invited to the gathering to speak about the role of grief as it related to the conference theme: "Dark Talk with Screeching Pines: Why Men Listen to Nature's Voices." The land was familiar to me, shaped by ancient glacial activity as it receded at the end of the last Ice Age. Having lived the first twenty-two years of my life in Wisconsin, I recognized the terrain immediately. It was in my body, and it spoke a familiar language.

The first thing I did when I arrived at the conference was to ask Miguel Rivera to introduce me to the Spirit of the Lake. Although the land was familiar to me, I was unknown to the place, and I wanted to step onto this land in a respectful way. We walked out on the pier and with tobacco and sweet words in Mayan, Lakota, Spanish, and English, we said hello and offered our greetings to this place. I brought greetings from the redwoods, the salmon people, madrone, and Douglas firs, the familiars from my coastal Northern California home. In beauty, it had begun.

The first night we stepped immediately into a ritual. It was clear to me that these men were carrying something deep and powerful. This was no mere conference but an established ritual ground whose intention is to dream and feed a new culture, one invigorated by ancient practices like ritual and renewed by the vital waters of myth and story, poetry, and singing. I was walking onto sacred ground. Some part of me felt deeply at home and grateful to find another place devoted to the mending of culture and the culture of mending men's souls.

I was asked to prepare a couple of talks that would be shared over the week. I realized I had a good deal of material on one topic and that it would fill the two times I would be invited to teach. My talk was called "A Beautiful and Strange Otherness." The title comes from a passage by the human biologist Paul Shepard that occurred in the course of an interview. He was asked what role the *others* played in our development as a species. The others here referred to the animals, plants, rivers, trees; the entire surrounding field that was the ongoing reflection we encountered for hundreds of thousands of years. Shepard's response was stunning, ending his thought with a sentence that has captivated me ever since I first read it many years ago. He said, "The grief and sense of loss, that we often attribute to a failure in our personality, is actually a feeling of emptiness where a beautiful and strange otherness should have been encountered."[40]

As is always the case when I share that quote, there is an immediate request to repeat it slowly as everyone scrambles for pen and paper. After I shared the passage, I said, "We could spend the rest of this gathering metabolizing the gravity of this one sentence."

The weight carried by this phrase astonishes me. We were meant to have a lifelong engagement with a beautiful and strange otherness. It was meant to be an ongoing presence, not an exception or something that we capture on our cameras while on vacation in Yellowstone or by watching it on the Nature channel. Shepard spoke adamantly and repeatedly about how the others shaped us and made us human; how the lessons of coyote and rabbit, mouse, and hawk taught us core values and how to live here in a sustainable way. Animal images were the first to appear in recesses and cave paintings, the first to be conjured in myths and tales. Their ways were integral not only to our survival but to the very shaping of our souls.

Now, in the shortest wisp of a moment, the perennial conversation has been silenced for the vast majority of us. There are no daily encounters with woods or prairies, with herds of elk or bison, and no ongoing connection with manzanita or scrub jay. The myths and stories about the exploits of raven, the courage of mouse, and the cleverness of fox have fallen cold. The others have retreated and have essentially vanished from our attention, our minds, and our imaginations. *What happens to our soul life in the absence of the others?* Shepard says that what emerges is a grief-laden emptiness. How true. He was wise, however, to recognize our tendency to attribute the emptiness to a "failure in our personality."

Nearly every day in my practice, I hear someone talk about feeling empty. But what if this emptiness is more akin to what Shepard is suggesting? What if what we are experiencing is a deep silence, a prolonged absence of birdsong, the scent of sweetgrass, the taste of wild huckleberries, the cry of the red-tailed hawk, or the melancholy call of the loon? What if this emptiness is the great echo in our soul of what it is we expected and did not receive?

We are born, wrote psychiatrist R. D. Laing, as Stone Age children.[41] Our entire psychic, physical, emotional, and spiritual makeup was shaped in the long evolutionary sweep of our species. Our inheritance includes an intimate and permeable exchange with the wild world. It is what we expected. Ecopsychologist Chellis Glendinning calls this original enfoldment in the natural world the *primal matrix*.[42] We were entangled, embedded in this matrix of life, and knew the world and ourselves *only* through this perception. It was an unmediated intimacy with the living world with no trace of separation between the human and the more-than-human world.

What was once a seamless embrace has now become a breach, a tear in our sense of belonging in the world. This rip in the fabric of our belonging is what Glendinning calls our "original trauma."[43] This trauma carries with it all the recognizable symptoms associated with this psychic injury: chronic anxiety, dissociation, distrust, hypervigilance, disconnection, as well as many others. We are left with a profound loneliness and isolation that we rarely acknowledge. It is as if we have completely normalized our condition. And yet, this feeling of separation profoundly affects the range of our reach into the world, the ways we participate in the landscape and sense our allegiance with the living world. Our soul life diminishes, flickers dimly, and rather than feeling a kinship with the entire breathing world, we inhabit and defend a small shell of a world, occupying our daily life with what linguist David Hinton calls the "relentless industry of self."[44]

Sigmund Freud recognized the reduction in our life that accompanies the process of enculturation. He wrote,

> Originally the ego includes everything, later it separates off an external world from itself. Our present ego-feeling is, therefore, a shrunken residue of a much more inclusive—indeed all embracing—feeling which corresponded to a once intimate bond between the ego and the world around it.[45]

We did not come here to be a shrunken residue of a formerly intimate life. This "beautiful and strange otherness" was also meant to be seen in one another's eyes. We too are meant to embody a vivid and animated life, to live close to our wild souls, our wild bodies and minds. We were meant to dance and sing, play, and laugh unselfconsciously, tell stories, make love, and take delight in this brief but privileged adventure of incarnation. The wild within and the wild without are kin, the one enlivening the other in a beautiful tango.

When we pause and allow our separation from the living earth to rise, we feel the "grief and sense of loss" that begins Shepard's ending response. When we open ourselves and take in the sorrows of the world, letting them penetrate our insulated hut of the heart, we are both overwhelmed by the grief of the world and, in some strange alchemical way, reunited with the aching, iridescent body of the planet. We become acutely aware that there is no "out there"; we share one continuous presence, one skin. Our suffering is mutually entangled, the one with the other, as is our healing.

On those nights when the skies are clear, my wife and I sit outside and let our eyes fall into the bowl of darkness. Wrapped in the blanket of night, we take in the beauty of Andromeda, Cassiopeia, and Albireo, feeling the larger home to which we belong. To come home is to remember our birthright; it is to recall that we are all indigenous to this stunning and wild world with its rumbling storms and lapis seas. Whatever fiction we ingested from a society that says we are separate from this animate world, we are, in fact, completely entangled with the beautiful and strange otherness that surrounds us. Our home is here, nestled with pine boughs and crows' wings, rambunctious otters, and rolling waves. Becoming attuned to this way of perceiving the earth is at the heart of what we are called to remember.

AN APPRENTICESHIP WITH SLOWNESS.   To notice these bonds of connection, however, we need to be moving in a way that is in accord with the rhythm of the soul. We need to move at what my mentor Clarke Berry called "geologic speed." The first

move we can make to help restore our connection with the beautiful and strange otherness is to recall the soul's primal rhythm.
This rhythm was established over hundreds of thousands of years
when we walked the earth. Our senses and minds were synchro-
nized to streams and night skies, to times around the fire, to the
long, patient wait of the hunter, and to listening to stories told by
elders. We moved slowly and drank in the entire spectrum of life
through our bodies. We need to take up an *apprenticeship with
slowness* and remember this ancient mode of being.

Slowing down offers us an opportunity to establish bonds of
intimacy with those around us—partners, children, and friends—
and out into the wider terrain of the beautiful and strange otherness. Imagine creating a friendship with a birch tree, a raven,
or a stone. Let something capture your attention, call to you, and
engage you in an extended conversation until you and this other
become entangled. Become good friends rooted in the practice of
familiarity and repetition. It takes time and repeated exposure
to know another. I know when I walk through certain woods,
how good it feels to come upon a familiar tree that I immediately recognize as an old friend, and we step into one another's
embrace and sit for a while in a restful silence, falling deeper into
our conversation.

UNCENTERING THE HUMAN.   The practice of entering into
the mind of another is what I call *uncentering the human*. This is
an ancient practice and an invitation to encounter the inner life of
the beautiful and strange otherness.

This is the second move we can make to connect with the wild
otherness that abounds around us. Whereas psychology encourages us to get centered, the wild soul wants to experience the
multicentric world in which we live and breathe. To do so is to
return to a vibrant intimacy with the world. This is an amazing

thought. What if our confidence was not based on some sense of personal power but more truly on the depth of intimacy we have with the animals, plants, and trees that inhabit the watersheds around our homes? What if our sense of confidence came from letting the ambling bear, the jumpy towhee, and the curving arc of a feather touch our inner world, reminding us that we are part of it all?

Soul Work

Let yourself recall some particular place, some presence that has been with you all your life. In your mind, walk around it, under it, above it, touch it, and breathe in its scent. Come to know this other in a new way. After you feel you have fully contacted it, let your attention slip inside it and become this other looking back at you. This totemic shift in awareness was something remarkably familiar to our ancestors and offered an extended experience of identity. Notice how you feel. Be as particular as you can, feeling the contours and movements of this being. And when you are ready, slip off this coat and come back to the one you recognize as yourself. Spend some time writing down what you encountered.

When we loosen the tight collar of civilization and step into the "culture of wildness,"[46] as storyteller Martin Shaw calls it, we recall the mutability of the self. We are part wolverine, part samba, part oak savanna. We come into the wider and wilder reach of our souls as we feel our branches stretching toward the sun, our roots penetrating the dark and mysterious soil. We feel ourselves as raindrops seeping into the dry ground. Our inheritance is this shapeshifting, storytelling, song-singing existence that we occupy for a short while. When we uncenter our lives and feel ourselves falling into the embrace of the world, we remember our greater life, the one brimming with aliveness and connection. It is here, on this outcropping of awareness, that the beautiful and strange otherness turns and looks back into our eyes. We shiver at this gaze, reminded that that same wildness is in us. Our identity widens and we once again find ourselves with talons and beak, fur and claws, and taking in sunlight through a hundred thousand tongues of green. We remember dancing around the firelight, singing songs, and telling stories, ritually honoring this ancient bond between us and the beautiful and strange otherness.

DRINKING THE TEARS OF THE WORLD. How can we fail to love this achingly beautiful world when we are so completely jumbled together with it all? It is our myopia, our species-centric blindness that cuts us off from the actual world. To love this world, however, is to also know sorrow. Our grief is intimately connected to how far we allow our love to reach into the world. Think of those Indigenous tribes willing to fight to the death to protect their homelands from being destroyed by mining or oil companies. They know their lives are inseparable from the animals, plants, rivers, spirits, and ancestors of their lands. Our love was also meant to spill out into the world, into the forests, the rivers, and cloud banks. It was not meant to congeal in a single person or even a single species. When this happens—when the arc between our bodies and the great body of the earth breaks—we fall into an attachment disorder of epic proportions, and everything suffers. Grief work is the third way we restore our bond with the world we inhabit.

The good news is we are supremely crafted to feel kinship with this breathing world. We are giant receptor sites for taking in the blue of the sky, the taste of honey, the caress of a lover, the scent of rain. Paul Shepard said we are more like a pond surface than a closed system: We are permeable, exchanging the vibrancy of wind, pollen, color, and fragrance. Life moves into us and through us like a breeze, affecting us and shaping us into a part of the terrain. We are inseparable from all that surrounds us. To mend the attachment disorder, we simply have to step out of our isolated room of self and into the wider embrace that awaits each of us. When we do, something magical happens. As we build our capacity for transparency and allow the world to enter us, our feelings of love blossom and an erotic leap occurs, bringing everything close to our heart. David Hinton writes in *Hunger Mountain*,

> I become broken clouds drifting frontier passes, Star River, . . . chrysanthemums and clotted dark. . . . I wander the changing forms of my unborn identity, and with each new form, I am more myself than ever. . . . I become winged sky and the talon-torn kill caught in the open fields of snow, warm meat I tear from sinew and bone slice by slice, kill I leave among wing-prints when I flap away downslope into an early-winter thermal, all sky again bearing taut, well-fed wings up into open sky.
>
> My heartbeats sound like dried grasses in gusty wind, like wing-beats and snowfall, like silent hunger-stares and pulsar, pulsar, pulsar. Heartbeat like footfall, silence, and shelling, like cosmic background microwave radiation, wingbeat, and snowmelt trickle-down ten-thousand-foot granite, shrapnel cries and silence, pulsar, dried grasses, my heartbeat heartbeat heartbeat.[47]

Hinton goes on from there, but his words give a glimpse into the larger Self that awaits us when we greet the beautiful and strange otherness. Our loneliness subsides and our feelings of exile wane. Imagine this level of belonging when pulsars and chromosomes are all weaving themselves through you and are you. There is no sentimentality in his words, however. They include death and grief, war, and hunger. It is all there as need be, and yet, we can feel the confidence that arises from such a wide reach of inclusion.

ENTERING THE STOREHOUSE OF MYTH.   A fourth pathway leading us back to the tracks of the beautiful and strange otherness is through the sensuous world of story and myth. Here, spirit horses and shaggy bears of desire move through our inner landscape. In this craggy wilderness of the soul, we wrestle with longing and loneliness, power and love, danger, and surprise meetings with strange allies. Our interior story merges with the great stories of all cultures, and we see how these deep streams come from a shared ocean of experience. The myths of the world emerge from the earth, from the great fertile ground beneath our feet. Becoming familiar with this rich storehouse of wisdom helps us feel our kinship with the wild earth and the deep rivers of culture.

We are being asked to dream, or more accurately, to become receptive to the dreaming Earth and hear the lingering echoes of ways of being that are latent in our psychic lives. We are completely designed for a life of soul and community, that twining trail through the thicket of intimacy and sovereignty. At times we must crawl on our hands and knees to recover the trail, but it is there, rooted in body and psyche, anchored by ancestors and the land—those perennial roots that hold us close to one another and to the singing soil. The most encouraging news is that we are not alone; we are surrounded by quivering aspens and the invisible hands of deep-time ancestors. We possess a secret, wild language, living stories and songs that carry love and remind us of the vast landscapes of beauty that live in us.

We are rooted to place, to soil, to brambles and oaks, to the stories that have risen out of the night mist around an ancient fire, told by the old ones who no longer inhale the sweet scent of smoke or sage. To remember our eternal bond with this beautiful and strange otherness is to recall our deep-time heritage, our mythic inheritance that is embedded in bone and breath. We become a burrowing badger of belonging, nosing our way into the soil, nuzzling the ground with sharp claws and an instinctual knowing that is determined to claim what is ours. The beautiful and strange otherness that Shepard calls us to encounter is within us and around us. Slow down, uncenter and forget about yourself for a moment, let the world find you, love what is nearby, share your grief with others, say thank you, learn the stories from where you live and from where your ancestors came, be a wee bit wild in your imagination, and come home.

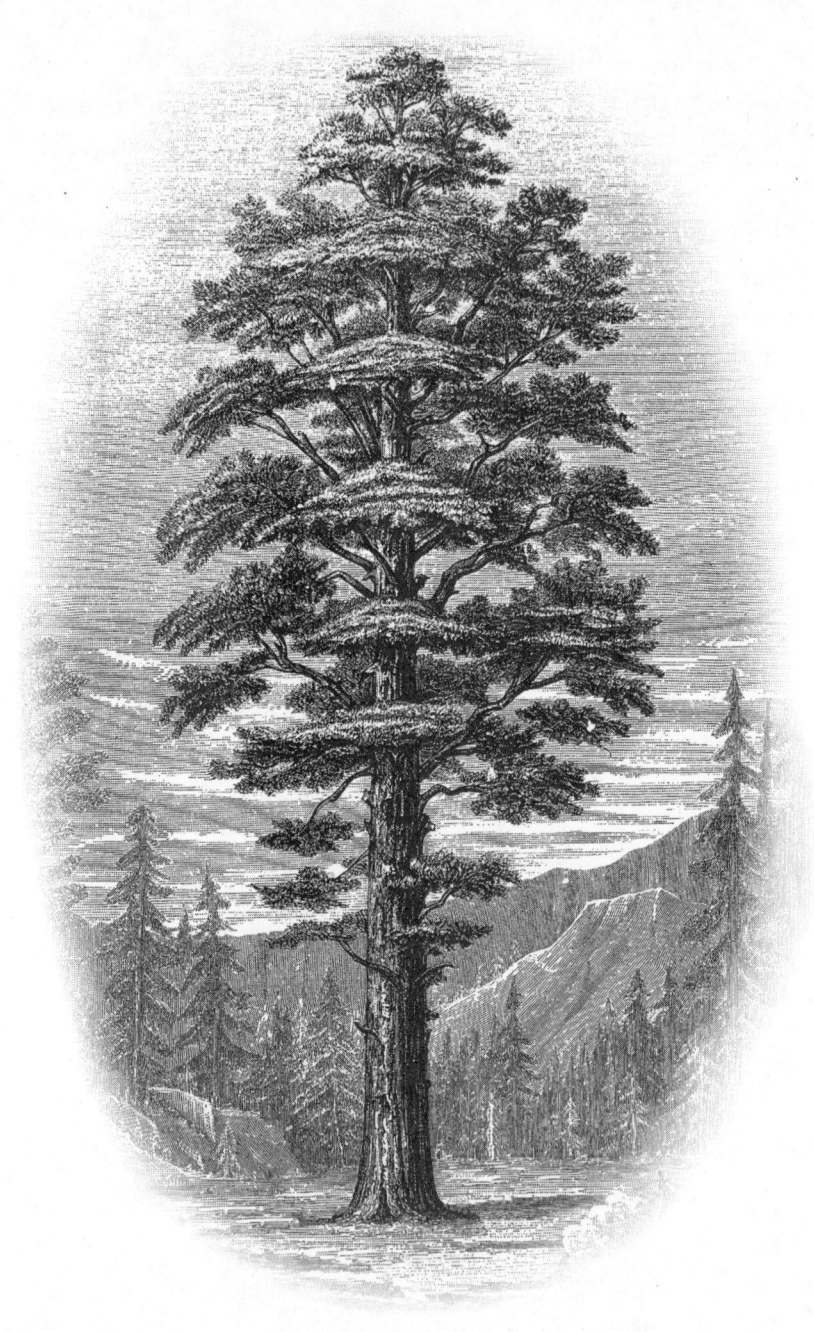

Fourteen

Redwood Speech, Watershed Prayers

The Erotics of Place

PLACE, TO INDIGENOUS CULTURES and the indigenous soul, is a living presence. Familiar watering holes, majestic mountains, sacred groves of trees, painted rocks, and caves where initiations were held added another dimension to life that is quite foreign to modern consciousness. To live within a sentient geography is to find oneself embedded in a rich and engaging terrain, a land that speaks. To our ancestors, and many Indigenous cultures today, the landscape was another voice, a territory imbued with mystery and power. What this offered was another way to encounter the sacred and to enliven the imagination. This fertile exchange between place and psyche established a bond with the land, which, in turn, created an ethos of respect for the land. When the ground holds value, when it is the dwelling place of the spirits and the ancestors, when magic swirls through the canyons and across the plains, the relationship between the people and the land becomes sacramental.

Place is sensual, particular, and felt as a presence offering itself to us for connection and spiritual sustenance. In traditional cultures, specific and revered places were saturated with stories, the ground filled with mythological rumblings; for example, the well-known storylines found in the landscape in the Dream-time myths of the Aboriginal peoples of Australia. Likewise, the

Western Apache in Arizona can name hundreds of sites where events took place "in the before time." To their ancestors, these pathways marked the ways of survival. They led to water and food sources, but even more, they also provided a palpable way of encountering the sacred through geography. To know the world this way, as a living icon, is to know in your body that you are walking upon holy ground. The Aboriginal peoples knew this quality as *djang*. James Cowan explains what this word meant:

> For them *djang* embodies a special power that can be felt only by those susceptible to its presence. In this way my nomad friends are able to journey from one place to another without ever feeling that they are leaving their homeland. What they feel in the earth, what they hear in the trees are the primordial whispers emanating from an ancient source. And it is this source, linked as it is to the Dreaming, that they acknowledge each time they feel the presence of the *djang* in the earth under their feet.[48]

Two days after my fortieth birthday I made my way to Armstrong Woods in Guerneville, a small town located about ten miles from the Pacific Ocean in Northern California. The town is situated on the Russian River, a beautiful waterway that begins some ninety miles to the north. From every perspective, you see the tall ones, the redwoods that tower above the valley floor, and during the winter these trees draw an amazing amount of water out of our storms. The town was named after George Guerne, a man who made his mark in the timber industry late in the 1800s. At that time, great stands of redwoods covered most of this area. Now, these woods, set aside as a nature preserve by Colonel James Armstrong in the 1870s, are one of the last remaining old-growth redwood groves in Sonoma County.

It had been raining hard for the previous few days and on this day the rains persisted. I had been planning this pilgrimage for a long time, and when I woke that morning the heavy rains disappointed me. I lay in bed for a while, unsure of what to do, but finally, I decided I had to go anyway. I gathered my gear and got in my truck for the drive to Armstrong. It poured all during the forty-minute journey to my destination.

When I pulled into the parking lot of the woods, it was deserted. The heavy weather had made a visit unappealing to others and so I had the old ones to myself. These trees, *Sequoia sempervirens*, are among the oldest living beings on the planet. They can grow over three hundred feet high and live for more than two thousand years. I came to a stop and turned off the truck. The moment I did, the rain stopped, and the sun appeared.

I got out of the truck and made my way through puddles and mud to the trailhead. Since it was late January, the air was cold, and the mist was high in the treetops, adding to the sudden brilliance and beauty of the day. The ground was saturated, and I had to make my way slowly down the path. The fragrance in the woods was musty, earthy, and rich with the smell of decay and growth, both at the same time. Each tree carried a profusion of jeweled droplets suspended from its branches. I came to one old giant known as the Parson Jones Tree, and gazed up toward its peak. Some three hundred feet high, out of my sight, it broke into the open. But down here at its base, I was the recipient of the most exquisite shower of gems. Each drop that fell from the tree carried the sun's light, came to the body of the earth pulled by the force of gravity, and offered itself to the earth as a blessing. I was mesmerized for a long time, drinking in the beauty of this combination of water and light. In deep gratitude, I reached out to touch the skin of this elder. Still, I knew I had to continue on, not knowing what I was searching for.

Deeper into the woods I went, enjoying the profound silence that the woods offered to me on that day. Even the birdlife was subdued. The occasional blue jay announced its presence with a loud bark, but other than the sound of water running in the creek beds, I was walking in silence.

At one point in my sauntering, I came to a redwood with one of the familiar natural openings often featured in pictures of these trees, openings deep enough to enter and stand inside, like a natural cave in the tree trunk. I felt moved to do so now. I stepped down a foot or so to the inner forest floor and stood there surrounded on three sides by the living membrane of this enormous presence. In this stillness, where only my breathing was audible, I heard another voice. Clearly and distinctly the voice said, "I am the Buddha." I waited quietly and heard the words repeated. "I am the Buddha. This is the dharma, and this is your sangha."

I recognized the words and their meanings. I myself had not spent much time studying Buddhist teachings but was aware of these specific terms. The Buddha was the teacher, the dharma was the teaching, and the sangha was the community that protected the student and provided the student with support and spiritual encouragement. I could only surmise that these words were coming from this ancient redwood. This old one *was* the Buddha, *was* the teacher; the forest and its complex interplay of kingdoms and phyla, species, and families were the teaching; and the community of sorrel and ferns, bay laurels, Douglas firs, and redwoods, creeks and stones, mushrooms, and lichen, live oaks, and blue jays were indeed my spiritual community.

I stood motionless to see if the message would be continued. I finally responded and said that I understood the message. Despite the brevity of this redwood's speech, it was profound. I had never heard nature speak so directly. I had had moments of intuition or images that conveyed a meaningful exchange but nothing this tangible. And so, I stood a long time in the darkness of the tree, within this great being's body, feeling as though I was wrapped within its essence.

For the next few days, I thought about this encounter. This redwood's speech was so intelligent. Somehow, in some way, it knew to use those exact words. I say that because I am so quick to question the legitimacy of mysterious messages from the spirit world, particularly experiences that are outside the familiar. When the tree chose to speak to me in those words—"Buddha," "dharma," and "sangha"—it forced me to recognize that the origin of this thought was outside my own consciousness because I would never have used those terms to speak to myself. That thought sent me into a period of wondering about the link between the outer world and myself, a link that I previously thought was less definitive. However, this experience revealed to me that the passage between outer and inner was more porous than I had known or than I had been led to believe. Perhaps I am known by the outer world in ways that I had not permitted myself to imagine before.

What was equally important, however, was the event itself and the teaching it carried for me. For far too long we have been detached from nature, from the particulars of the world and her ways of instructing us in how to be a part of the mosaic of life. This knowing is what made our ancestors human in the best sense of the word. "Human" shares the same root origins as "humus," meaning "of the earth." Despite all our fantasies of transcendence, resurrection, and ascension, despite all our technologies that separate us and insulate us from the sensual world, we are creatures of this earth, and our substance is informed by the speech of the world.

I go back often to visit this redwood tree with a feeling of friendship and a growing familiarity, realizing that I am hungry for a language that conveys the truth of our bond with the world.

Traditional cultures rarely had words that specified generalities like "tree." Instead, they had ways of identifying an individual presence—a specific tree—in the woods. This language of particularity generates a much more sensuous relationship due to the simple fact that naming requires knowing. Conversely, I think of how little time we spend in the woods, along riverbanks, in the hills and mountains. These places have become our vacation destinations, but we seldom develop and nurture relationships with them that can evolve and endure through time. How can we come to know the individualities that exist in the world without time and patience, without attention and relationship? It may be that much of what the soul suffers from is related to this severing of its vital connection with the animate world.

When we create an intimate relationship with a place, it becomes for us a refuge. This communion offers us a more thorough expression of our innate complexity. Our entire biological structure is designed for engagement with the world. Every sense organ is a gateway for encounter, and through this exchange, we achieve a greater definition of who we are. The senses are the means by which our bond with the world is consummated and made sacramental. The radical genius William Blake said, "Man has no Body distinct from his Soul for that call'd Body is a portion of Soul discern'd by the five Senses, the chief inlets of Soul in this age."[49] It is through the blood and sensuality of this flesh that we become incarnate. Till then, till we know that our place is in the world and that our bodies emerged from this earth, we cannot know who we are.

Language too is rooted to place, to the land. Our imagination is shaped by landscape and topography. Language can either reflect the abundance, the richness of our belonging to a complex and vital community of life or it can reflect a poverty born of exile.

I am enthralled with the language of Indigenous people. Not only does it carry beauty in its sound, but also the words themselves reflect an unbroken arc between the speaker and their surroundings. In many of these languages, there is no dichotomy, no separation that strands the human in a point of separation as a cold observer. When a Diné or an Inuit man or woman speaks, the cosmos is imminent, not abstracted or referenced. There is seldom the separation between subject and object that we find in our English language. This is hard for us to comprehend, but it is invaluable for us to know that there are other ways of knowing the world. For example, the San people possess an onomato-poetic language that is as close to the sensual world as possible, its cadences mirroring the sounds of the living earth—rain, bird-calls, animal sounds. The complex clicks of their speech mimic the rhythms of the actual life around them so that they are constantly immersed in the surrounding terrain.

I feel deep grief when I think about how far we have deviated from the intimacy we once knew with the earth. Sitting here along the northern coast of California while my wife gathers sweetgrass, I see a tree with a golden ladder rising from its base. A fungus has emerged from this dying elder, an enormous Monterey pine, and this stairway arises from its decay, orchestrating a new beauty. The sun is illuminating the new growth, and it offers itself to me with a radiance that makes me think of Jacob and his celestial stairway.

I have been trying to place myself back into the world as if I could leave it! Yet spiritually that is what my culture has taught me to do. I carry deep conditioning shaped by two thousand years of images, stories, and ideals that renders life here on earth as some form of sentence to be commuted through death. We console ourselves about the deaths of those we love by saying that they are now in a better place. The earth is to be transcended: heaven is the *better world* that will somehow make up for the pain and sorrow of time spent here, our *final reward*, as it were. I find this offensive and could never believe that the Jesus I know would have ever felt such contempt for the earth. This was the man who constantly referred to the earth, to her creatures, and to the growing things as examples in his teachings. This was the man who retreated to the wilderness on a number of occasions to gather himself back to himself. Nature, the wild, the world contained and held him.

The wild undoubtedly shaped our original words: imitations of animal sounds, wind, thunder, and the music of ocean and river. This lustrous blend of sounds quickened the imagination of our ancestors and, as I said earlier, even a cursory glance at tribal language reveals a richly textured, complex syntax of metaphor and imagery deeply imbued with the surrounding world. In the Amazon, for example, language is imbued with metaphors of the jungle to express a multitude of situations and aspects in the lives of the people. Jay Griffiths writes, "Metaphor is where language is most wild, spirited, and free, leaping boundaries, and it may be no surprise that Amazonian languages can be as matted and dense with metaphor as the forest is tangly with vegetation. The Amazon seems a place of boundless allusion, this unfenced wild, where meaning is twined within meaning; words couple and double, knotted together."[50] Our modern lexicon, however, reveals erosion in our formerly flowering language. We are now speaking in acronyms, and abbreviations, texting our words through phones. My feeling is that as our senses are deprived of the multiple cadences from a living world, so too does our language atrophy. We are left with bare rhetoric instead of a kind of speech that can bring us to tears or into symmetry with the many others with whom we share the world.

In a very real way, language and place are synonymous. Words reflect what we inhabit and where we dwell. Geologian and author Thomas Berry said that our imagination is only as rich as the diversity of the life around us. If we inhabit a terrain of microchips, cell phones, and video monitors, we speak two-dimensionally, abstractly because there is nothing sensual about these realities.

If, on the other hand, our daily round includes sunlight, fragrances from the green earth, songbirds, and tastes of berries picked from the bush, then our sensual minds stir, and the words become as richly textured as the terrain. Our language has an ecology, and it is as varied as the experiences it is given. Jay Griffiths speaks to this in her book *Wild: An Elemental Journey*: "All languages have long aspired to echo the wild world that gave them growth and many Indigenous peoples say that their words for creatures are imitations of their calls. According to phenomenologist Maurice Merleau-Ponty, language 'is the very voice of the trees, the waves, the forest.'"[51]

Oral traditions are metaphorical and creative, filled with rich imagery. Stories were held in memory, that is, *by heart*, and the wisdom was continuous from generation to generation. We have a challenging time memorizing our social security number let alone a phenologic account of a living system. What migrates when? What is ripe now? When do we relocate to the winter grounds? How do we prepare the acorns? How do we resolve conflict? How does one become a man or a woman? Stories were the carriers of this wisdom, and the words used to transport the stories were alive with meaning and significance.

I want to see our words jump off the ground and erupt from sensual earth, musty, humid, gritty. I want to taste words like honey, sweet and dripping with eternity. I want to hear words coming from my mouth and your mouth that are so beautiful that we wince with joy at their departure and arrival. I want to touch words that carry weight and substance, words that have shape and body, curve, and tissue. I want to feel what we say as though the words were holy utterances surfacing from a pool where the gods drink. What if our words could once again echo the larger reality of the sacred and not solely the world of economics? But that would take an act of remembrance, a slowing downward into a state of presence, awareness, and being. And this means being in the world. Enough of this talk that makes us strangers! I want to know I belong here. And if my words can say to you that I am a man of this earth, this particular piece of earth, then I will feel like I have arrived. My language must be redwood speech, watershed prayers, oak savanna, coupled in an erotic way with fog, heat, wind, rain, hills, sweetgrass and jackrabbits, wild iris, and ocean current. My land is my language and only then can my longing for eloquence be granted. Until then I will fumble and fume and ache for a style of speaking that tells you who I am.

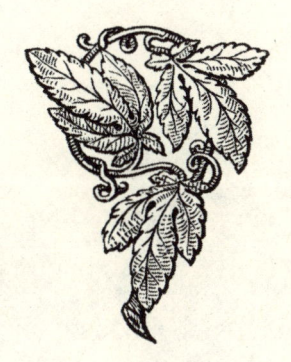

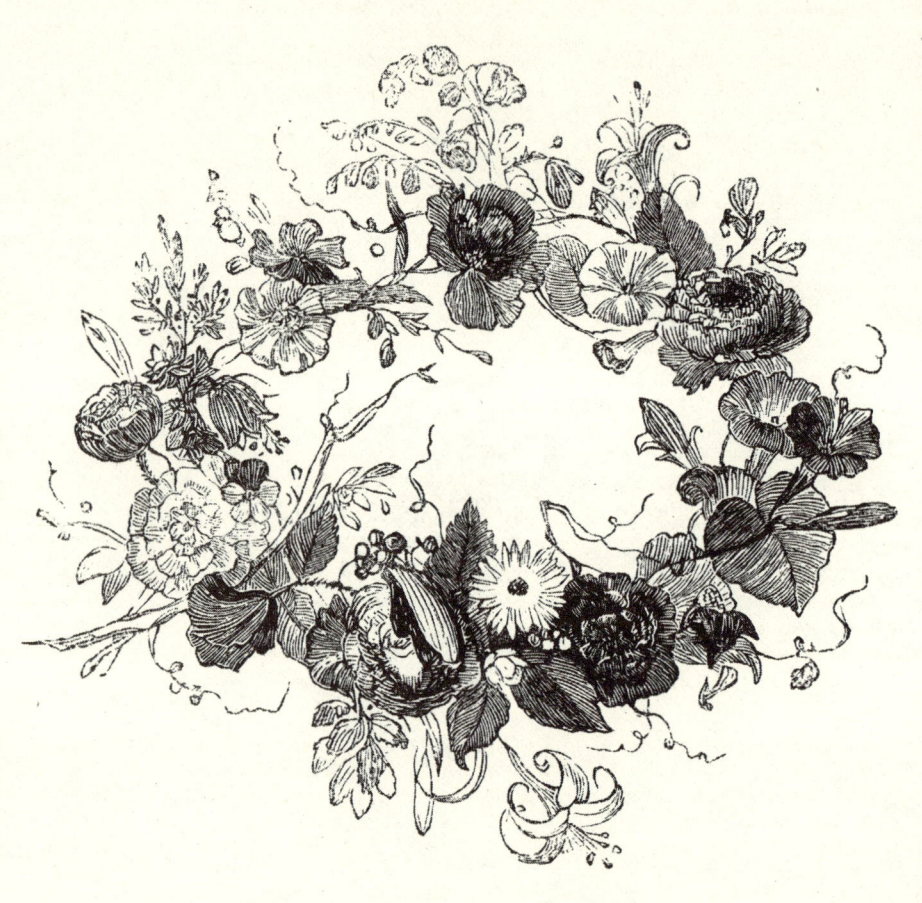

Fifteen

Gratitude for All That Is

THERE IS A TRADITION among the Native people of the Iroquois Confederacy that goes back more than a thousand years. It is known as the Thanksgiving Address. In the language of their people it is called *Ohen:ton Karihwatehkwen*, which translates to "Words Before All Else." The tradition involves the invocation of creation in a manner that extends thankfulness to all living things for their gifts to us. In this way, the people are brought into alignment with nature. This eloquent ritual practice places gratitude as the beginning point for any further matters. Words Before All Else. What if our daily practice were to include this deep-seated reverence for creation and acknowledge the never-ending flow of blessings that come our way? I remember Brother David Steindl-Rast saying, "It is not happiness that makes gratefulness, but gratefulness that makes happiness."[52]

Gratitude is a central value to the indigenous soul. It forms the very heart of a life rooted in the awareness and recognition that we truly live in a gifting cosmos. Our deep-time ancestors, and those remaining Indigenous cultures still living in the old ways, know that everything we need has been given to us. In the ecology of the sacred, our responsibility is to receive these blessings with gratitude. What is the proper response to a gift if not gratitude? This understanding formed the basic attitude of traditional people, and it is also readily recognized when we, too, turn our attention to this fundamental truth.

Gratitude furthers the soul and calls it forth into the world in an act of intimacy. The simple gesture of receptivity paired with the expression of thankfulness completes the arc that binds the soul and world together in communion. Doing so confirms our relatedness with the cosmos, and it is relationship that we are so in need of today. Our isolation and loneliness are in great part the consequence of forgetting to say thank you. This may sound simplistic, but it is true. We live in a completely interdependent world, and gratitude is the acknowledgment of this fundamental reality.

There is an old thought that says the strength of a community is reflected in the presence of generosity. In other words, the richness of the village is made visible by the expression of appreciation, recognition, and thankfulness for the ways the people support one another and the way the world holds the people together. It seems that we are bereft of such a unifying ingredient at this time. Rather than acknowledging the multiple layers of gifting that are offered to us, we focus more on lack, on what is missing. This is not some cynical move but a consequence of conditioning that continually references us back to what it is we do not have. Modernity keeps us hungry for more by turning our gaze toward absence. Psychology colludes in this as well by focusing primarily on what is wrong, what we did not get in childhood, and so on. This chronic feeling of not enough makes it difficult to register blessings and feel gratitude. It is our task to stay aware of what is being gifted here and now and to register the primary satisfactions that enrich our soul life, our emotional and bodily life. These are what make the moment thick with meaning and contentment: we have enough.

Gratitude is a spiritual responsibility. A grateful heart acknowledges and participates in the ongoing exchange with life. Gratitude is an act of faith, of trust in the ways of life. It is a confirmation that we are inextricably bound to each other thing in the cosmos. In this sense, it is a reflection of belonging. Another thought of Br. David's was that we can feel either grateful or alienated, but never at the same time. Gratefulness softens our sense of alienation. Our belonging is celebrated in thanksgiving, in full appreciation that we are both givers and receivers in the exchange of blessings.

How do we develop gratitude? The most fundamental practice is listening. This attentive move slows us down to the speed of life where we are more resonant with the movements of the world. By listening we can register in our bodies just how fluid this flow of blessings is in our lives. Think about that. The constancy of the sun, moon, and stars, the generosity of the rains, rivers, the earth, the abundant richness of birdsong, the fragrance of roses, wet streets after a downpour, the delectable sweetness of blackberries warm with the heat of the day, the luscious colors of fall, all are offered to us freely. When we listen and take in the astonishingly sensuous earth, we come awake to the thunderous beauty that surrounds us. We are inundated with the world pouring through every opening, and in this awareness, we recognize a fundamental truth: We are of the earth. In fact, as cosmologist Brian Swimme suggests, humans were put on earth to gawk. That is our cosmological destiny! To be astonished, amazed, and delighted in the intricate weavings of the cosmos is to listen fully, and to send out our sigh of appreciation is what is asked in return.

A second means by which we develop gratitude is through ritual. Ritual is the pitch through which our personal and collective voices are extended to the unseen dimensions of life, beyond the point of our minds, and into the realms of nature and spirit.

There are many opportunities for daily rituals that can drop us into a felt connection with life. Every meal we eat is a cosmological event. The renowned Buddhist monk and teacher Thich Nhat Hanh reminds us that through the practice of mindfulness, we become aware of the deep story within every meal. We are wedded to the cycles of sunshine and rain, the movements of microbes and root systems, the farmer and butcher, the animals and plants, and the grocery store clerk. The entire cycle that brings the morsel to our mouths is what we are ingesting and to behold that movement with gratitude is to sacralize the moment.

Our annual Gratitude for All That Is ritual is a beautiful gesture to the visible and invisible worlds. To communally send our prayers of thanksgiving into the world is a rich and verdant act. Our ritual is eloquent and simple. After building a gratitude shrine, we make our prayers and offer small gifts to the other world of tobacco, cornmeal, agates, or whatever has been brought. These gifts are offered in a small crawl-in grotto made of fir boughs and ferns where they are left overnight. In the morning, some children are asked to gather the offerings together and we then make our way singing across the grounds into the woods where a small opening is waiting to receive the gifts. At that time, the children that are there come forward and place handfuls of the offerings into the Mother's body and for that moment we are aligned with the rightness of our lives and the community. We have placed something back into her body in an act of recognition that everything we have comes from her. It is sweet medicine.

Gratitude is the other hand of grief. It is the mature person who welcomes both. To deny either reality is to slip into chronic depression or to live in a superficial reality. Together they form a prayer that makes tangible the exquisite richness of life in this moment. Life is hard and filled with suffering. Life is also a most precious gift, a reason for continual celebration and appreciation. To everything, as the old prophet said, there is a season. This is the time of giving thanks.

PART IV

❧

Closing Thoughts

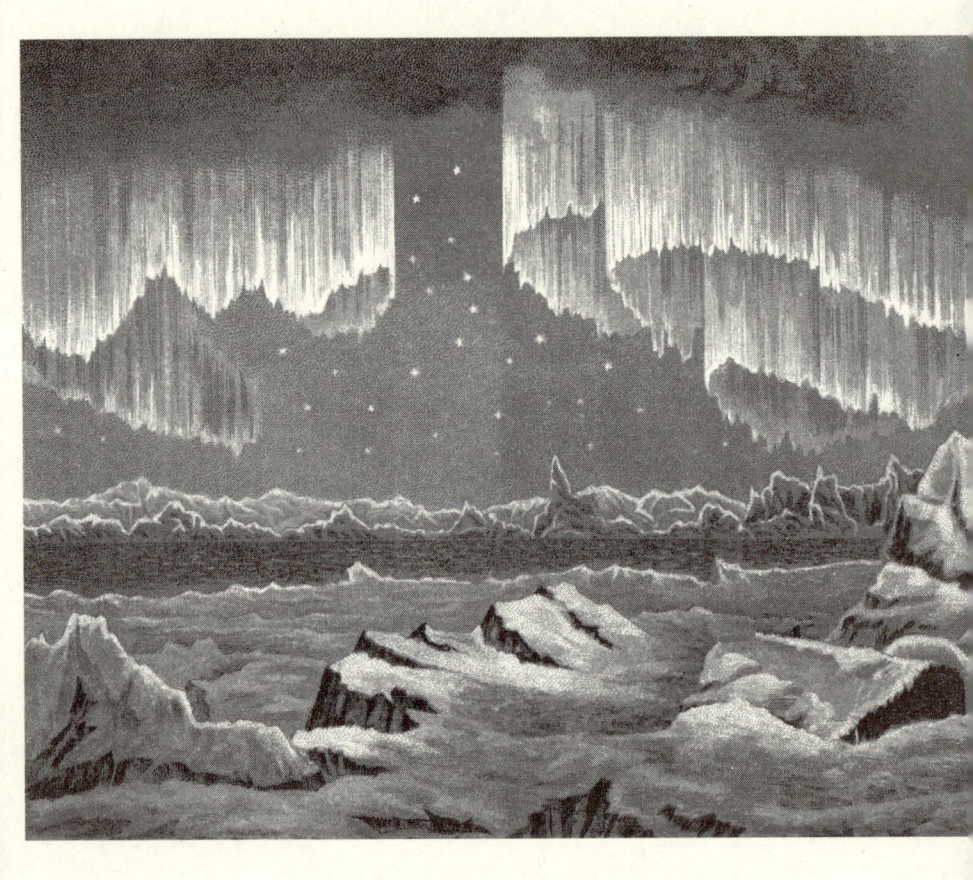

Sixteen

Medicine for the Long Dark

Dear friend,

Having you join me on this soul exploration in this season of descent has been a great gift. We feel the gravity of these times, the immense pull downward into the Long Dark. And yet, as we have seen, through the eyes of soul, this movement into the darkness is not filled with dread or panic but rather with a sense of expectancy, that within this cavern of night a sacred gestation is taking place. Still, we both know the period ahead of us will be difficult, the losses multiple, and the pathways ahead unknown. It is easy to feel anxious, panicked, and afraid, along with an almost crushing grief for the state of the world. It can feel overwhelming. So, how do we keep our little boat of self afloat? One question we must ask is: "What do we need to stay present and engaged and to keep our love moving into a world of radical uncertainty and change?" The world aches for our love, our affection, and our devotion. Our hearts need to be supported to keep the aperture of love open and flowing outward. We need robust medicine for the Long Dark.

I have been drawn to the idea of medicine for a long time. Every essay in this collection carries a thread of medicine that we can call upon, share with others, and that will support us in meeting the Long Dark with presence and care.

The word "medicine" evokes many associations. Most notably, we connect medicine with healing, curing, and fighting against viruses or pathogens. We witness the work of medicine to treat cancer, fight infections, and relieve physical ailments. I know many who have benefited from these various forms of medicine, as have I, and feel deep gratitude for their amazing capacities to ease suffering.

Medicine, seen from a soul perspective, carries other possibilities as well. There are soul medicines that heal our relationships with the earth, with our watersheds, and with our ancestors. There are soul medicines that repair shattered communities after trauma. On numerous occasions I have been called to bring the medicine of ritual into circles facing acute grief and loss. This is soul medicine.

A central quality of soul medicine is *resistance*, a protest against reducing the wide arc of our lives into a meager expression as we try to fit into the cultural demands for conformity. The soul resists such a flattening of our essential being. We came to participate fully and to display the soul's grandeur. Resistance is also found in the wider collective body, where we witness efforts to stop damages to villages, food sources, sacred sites, and the next generation from corporate incursions designed to extract resources from traditional lands. Think Standing Rock or the Black Lives Matter movement or removing dams along the Klamath River.

Another form of soul medicine is *remembering*. Recalling our deep-time inheritance helps us counter the layers of amnesia that have settled like silt upon us. To remember is to heal. To remember is to return and come back into a vital and engaged relationship with all our relations. More on this in the next section.

My friend, let me offer some initial thoughts on what a medicine bundle for the Long Dark might include. I have been sitting with this question for some time. I have found that this exploration is multilayered. We need a soul medicine that can fortify us during this challenging time. It's also important to recognize that we already carry medicine for the Long Dark. Most astonishingly, there is medicine to be found in the Long Dark. Let me explain.

The Medicine We Need for the Long Dark

Friendship and community are the first medicines we require in the Long Dark. Within friendship's embrace we find a deep and often abiding sense of belonging. These belongings grant shelter from the turbulent emotions that can arise amid uncertainty and loss. We need places of refuge. *Refugia* is a term I love. I first came upon it while reading *Great Tide Rising* by Kathleen Dean Moore, a wonderful writer and teacher from Oregon. In her book, she described that when scientists first explored the devastated landscape of Mount St. Helens following the massive volcanic eruption in 1980, they assumed it would not recover in their lifetimes. Thirty-five years later, however, they discovered life had found a way to return. In little spaces on the side of the mountain, the scientists came across lees shaped by fallen logs and rocks within which small ferns, voles, fir seedlings, and moss were found. Little pockets of life returning from the devastation. They called these small folds of new life *refugia*: "Places of safety where life endures."[53] This is such a beautiful image and metaphor for us to linger around. This is strong medicine for the Long Dark. This is soul medicine we can offer to ourselves and others. We can become a refugia.

Friendship and community come from our fellow humans, but also from the rich and varied more-than-human world of animals, trees, rivers, and moonlight. This extensive community of beings reminds us of our entanglement with all things and our broader home in the world.

One night, several years ago, I was heading to sleep filled with despair and dread over the state of things in our culture. As I was about to get into bed, something turned me around and guided me to one of my bookcases and I found my hand reaching for a collection of writings by Linda Hogan, a Chickasaw poet and elder. The book was *Dwellings: A Spiritual History of the Living World*. I randomly opened the book to the chapter "All My Relations." I realized, in that moment, that I had forgotten my kinship with the redwoods and fir, the lichen and ferns, the sorrel and night sky. When I brought them back to my attention, the despair lifted and a sense of ease entered my being. We cannot face the Long Dark without all of our relations.

Friendship is meant to be reciprocal, a mutual exchange of care, warmth, and attention. This truth tells us that any relationship of substance requires effort and nourishment. Friendship is always mutual. It is not something we simply receive; it is something we exchange. Over many decades, I have often noticed that our wounds around love keep us seeking places of belonging. At some point, in our movement toward adulthood, we must recognize that it is also our responsibility to create and become a place of belonging for others.

Friendship and community are protective. When we live within the folds of friendship, we can sense that whatever befalls us, we will be sheltered under the covering of community. We will not be left to fend for ourselves.

A second medicine that can help us engage the Long Dark is *imagination*. Imagination is rarely understood as central to our psychological lives. For the most part, imagination is seen as either wishful thinking or a waste of time. We emphasize the need to be practical and productive. All important, I know. Soul, however, revels in the undulations of the imaginal: the sensuous, spiraling, gyrating movements of images arising from the unseen world.

Carl Jung said that the psyche's primary activity is image-making. When we pause and notice, the images are there continuously. Through the ongoing generation of images, we are invited to sense our deeper lives and become receptive to the dreams of the soul and the earth. And isn't darkness the domain of dreams, mystery, gestation, and creation?

Imagination invites us to loosen our fixed sense of identity and allow a more porous experience to arise. In other words, our rigid definition of who we are begins to soften in the realm of the imaginal, when the separation between self and world is relaxed. Our choices and actions are affected by this reshaped terrain. Who are we in the dusk light of the Long Dark? Who might we become in our prolonged wandering in the unknown? We may come into a wider sense of self and feel our affinity with finch and laurel, sagebrush, and coyote. Image as a bridge. Image as a threshold to a richer sense of connection and affiliation. This extended aperture to our sense of self fortifies us as we uncenter ourselves and feel our kinship with all beings. We are large.

Imagination is also central to cultural renewal. It informs the gestures and practices made by the people to support the community. For example, the Dreamtime of the Aboriginal peoples of Australia. To these tribal cultures, the Dreaming is the real world; it is the world behind this one, upholding and sustaining the tangible, physical world. The rituals, songs, dances, songlines, paintings, and sacred sites necessary to maintain relations with the ancestors and spirit beings arose from the Dreaming. Participating in these practices, in turn, is what keeps the world alive. When we neglect and abandon the imaginal realm, the world corrodes and fades; the world loses its shine and beauty. All we need to do is look at modernity with its continual emphasis on progress, power, and profit to see the dimming effects on the shimmering world.

I trust you can see how vital the imagination is in facing the Long Dark. If there is no dream of the Earth, and if our capacities for imagination remain undeveloped, then we will not be able to receive and respond to the images as they are offered. We must listen and feel the dreaming Earth to keep our world green and vital. If we can, however, find our way back to the world of soul, sensing the innate aliveness present there, the world regains its psychic depths, its soul! I pray we dare to lean into the imagination and be stirred by the dream of the soul. I pray we can recover the medicine that dwells in the forest of the imagination.

A third medicine we can call upon as we move farther into the Long Dark is our *deep-time ancestral inheritance*. This is what I call the Trail on the Ground. During a time when the ordinary has been dislodged, we are not without markers and cairns that can show us a way of living that enables us to find steady ground, a sturdy heartbeat.

This inheritance returns us to the *commons of the soul*, what Jung called the "unforgotten wisdom at the core of the psyche."[54] Within this ancestral lineage is a storehouse of soul memory that recalls how to respond to the very conditions we are facing. We are not the first ones to face difficult times. And isn't that ancestral memory what we need in this prolonged season of darkness? Places where the craft of living culture can be remembered and developed. These deep-time memory echoes help us to attune to the movements and gestures needed during this time.

For all of us, there remains an immense reservoir of wisdom and survival that can help us find our way through the Long Dark. While we speak of the transgenerational transmission of trauma, we can also access the transgenerational transmission of courage, resilience, love, creativity, and strength. We are here because of the success of our ancestors. This is good news! Attending to this lineage gives us ballast, something reliable for us to lean on as things shift and change.

This deep-time memory reserve is often felt at our ritual gatherings. There have been several occasions when someone says, "I have never done anything like that before, but it felt oddly familiar" after a ritual. What is it in us that recognizes these moments as familiar? The archaic psyche, the "inner ancestor" as Michael Meade calls it, the "primal matrix" as Chellis Glendinning has named it, that senses this knowing. By whatever name, the ancestral lineage is within us, influencing our choices and ways of encountering the world. This deep resource is available to help all of us face the world with soul.

The Medicine We Bring to the Long Dark

We catch a glimpse of the medicine we bring to the Long Dark in an unexpected place. Surprisingly, it is nestled in the territory of our wounds. Not exactly the place we thought to look. So, with each successive encounter with our suffering, and as we work with our wounds, we slowly discern that something is hidden within the wound.

An idea from ancient Greece says, "In your wound is your genius." In other words, the wound brings us closer to the ground of soul. When we free ourselves from the excessive commentaries about our wounds being evidence of our unworthiness, we begin to see how the wound has acted as a catalyst, drawing us into the eros of darkness. Here we encounter vulnerability, sorrow, heartache, longing, affection, tenderness, surrender, nightmares, grace, intimacy, touch, and listening.

Our wounds keep us circling soul, around the depths of our "secret inside flesh." This gravitational pull draws us into a persistent relationship with our weakness and vulnerability, and with what is most intimate about our interior lives. Soul has an ongoing interest in the *inferior*. By inferior I am not making a moralistic comment but acknowledging the many pieces of soul life that have been rejected by dominant society. We live in a heroic culture, so what is often considered inferior are the parts of us that don't measure up to the image of the hero. Consequently, weakness, need, sadness, fear, insecurity, and many others are frequently pushed to the edges of our lives. Personally, and culturally, we find soul at the margins.

When we extend this thought to the Long Dark, the world also speaks to us through its symptoms and wounds. In our psyches, we register the depression, anxiety, pollution, trauma, violence, fear, and unrestrained consumption that is occurring in the collective field. As much as we would like to think that we are immune from these matters, our bodies tell us differently. Now, the patient is the planet, and her troubles are showing up in our lives, our therapy, our dreams, and our relationships. Through her afflictions, the soul of the world is drawing us into her depths. The fixed separation between inner and outer is rapidly dissolving.

The material in the vessel is essential. Alchemy declares that the work of soul-making, of generating the pearl of great price, begins in the discarded matter, the *putrefactio*, the decaying and dying parts of us; and by extension, the same principle holds for the wider culture. What has been collectively denied, neglected, or rejected becomes the beginning of the alchemical work.

How we approach our wounds largely determines whether we are able to recognize the medicine latent in the wound. If we approach with judgment and contempt, there will be no revelation about medicine. If we come to this tender territory with reverence, then, as John O'Donohue said, "Great things will approach us."

Illness Calls Forth the Medicine, an Ancient Call-and-Response

As we ripen and mature, and hopefully the ideology of perfection fades, we discern how our wounds sensitized us to the medicine we are asked to offer the community. We discover how our places of pain, trauma, shame, and suffering were the vessels within which our medicine was given shape. This is a profound soul move, an alchemical move that places our shame, traumas, and betrayals within the vessel for slow transmutation into medicine. This is not an easy process, but an essential move by which our soul calling finds its way into the world.

I think of my own experience of shame and how debilitating this wound was for me for decades. Over time, and after many attempts to rid myself of this unwelcome guest, I finally began to turn toward the shame and meet it with warmth. I slowly came to see how the shame had worked me over decades into someone who could sit with others in the most twisted places in their being. Shame taught me about the depths and the vulnerability of feeling outside and unworthy of connection. Only by welcoming the wound was I able to see the medicine latent in the suffering. True alchemy.

The slow digestion of our wounds, the gradual enclosure of our suffering within the container of compassion, yields the medicine the village needs. Vesseling the wound! The slow titration of trauma/wounds into blessings. This is the medicine of *compassion* for ourselves and the collective body. We all know suffering and we are all worthy of compassion.

The second medicine we develop in our interior world is our capacity to *turn toward* fear, grief, and anxiety. This is a central psychological task for each of us. As we turn toward the suffering, we simultaneously separate from it. This move is crucial. Only then can we grant our pain sufficient compassion to allow it to heal. Only then can we offer the spaciousness that enables us to see our wounds as inevitable and, in some strange way, necessary.

The ambient field surrounding us now is humming with fear, sorrow, anxiety, and a generous helping of dread. Our capacity to *turn toward* these difficult energies is an invitation that arises from the wound; to become immense. I remember working with a young woman at the Cancer Help Program. During one of our conversations, she said that she was filled with terror about how her cancer would impact her life. She was young and just starting her married life and suddenly she was dealing with a life-threatening cancer. As we sat together, I asked her if she had ever, in her lifetime, encountered something she might describe as sacred. She paused and then related a story of being in a sweat lodge where she experienced a profound connection with her ancestors.

"Is that woman who felt that deep connection with the ancestors bigger than the terror?" I asked her.

"Absolutely," she said.

"That is how big you need to be right now. You need to be able to get your arms around everything that is arising, including the fear," I said.

In that moment, she was able to turn toward these tender parts of herself and grant them shelter.

The Medicine We Find in the Long Dark

In the Long Dark, we find a different way of knowing, one rooted in soul. If we remember the injunction to approach with reverence, we might sense the holiness that dwells in the darkness. This is a holiness nested in what Buddhist teacher Deborah Eden Tull calls the "luminous darkness,"[55] what poet David Whyte calls a "deep but dazzling darkness,"[56] and what Buddhist teacher and anthropologist Joan Halifax calls a "fruitful darkness."[57]

We are taken into the underworld, a sightless terrain where we are asked to see through different means, to gain a second sight.

What do we discover in this shadowed terrain? The medicine of *entanglement*, the web of relationship that gathers everything together: hillsides, cloud banks, forests. We find our shared roots that connect us with the *anima mundi*, and by extension, the heart of matter—the sensual, erotic field of aliveness. Following Jung, the deeper we go down into psyche, our sense of individual uniqueness retreats farther and farther into darkness. We become increasingly part of the collective. Jung writes, "The body's carbon is simply carbon. Hence, at bottom, the psyche is simply world."[58] In some very real way, we are as much world as self! As much communal as personal. Our loneliness is eased when we sense our extensive entanglement with all that is. As we feel intimacy with the world, our compassion grows. This is a natural extension.

Other medicines we find in the Long Dark are the twin qualities of *patience* and *rest*. Patience grants us a pause, a slowing downward, which we know from our exploration of repetition is essential for coming into the rhythms of soul. This spaciousness can welcome all that is touched by grief, fear, longing, and more. Patience is a gathering place for all that has come into our embrace during our long walk in darkness.

We can't force things in the darkness. The legitimacy of our heroic efforts feels empty in the shadowed terrain of the Long

Dark. This is a place of waiting, silence, vigil, and alert witness-ing. Something is here, a vital and animating presence is here, in the darkness. Patience encourages us to become receptor sites for the emerging dream of the Earth. This is holy work.

And rest. To stop, rest, and disengage from the mania of pro-ductivity, achievement, and speed, the primary values of our daylit world, is a subversive act. We rarely stop to rest. So, we never truly restore or renew. Many of us feel exhausted. Rest. Restore. Renew.

In the soul medicine of the Long Dark, we find not only per-mission to rest and slow down but also encouragement. It's in the place of rest that dreaming can occur. It's also where we begin to feel the intimate movements of soul. Soul is subtle so we need to move at a rhythm slow enough to become attuned to her emerg-ing mystery.

This is what we need in the Long Dark. This is what we bring to the Long Dark. This is what we find in the Long Dark. The idea I'm trying to share with you, my friend, is that we are not without medicine. We have what we need to navigate the long season ahead. We have the resources. We have access to our gifts. We have friendship and community to lean into when need be. We are all carriers of medicine and there are many other forms of medicine available. Beauty, laughter, awe, nature, creativity, play, and many others are all vital forms of support to help us walk steadily during the Long Dark.

We have entered a liminal terrain where everything is chang-ing. We don't know what will happen. We do know there's med-icine available to respond to the challenges we will be facing. We are being ripened to become a place of shining darkness, a point of combustion, of incandescence. We will still know joy, passion, delight, and wonder in the Long Dark. The decades ahead will not be a steady pall of gray and shadow. The world will need our affection and warmth, our outrage and kindness. Let us become capable of generating a living culture once again. Let us dream of a wild earth, teeming with life and richness. We are not bereft. We are not alone. We are part of this dreaming Earth. There are many forms of sweet soul medicine.

I hope this long missive was helpful to you. There will be much to metabolize over the coming years and decades. Knowing that we have access to multiple forms and styles of medicine is reassuring. I look forward to continuing our conversation. In the meantime, I wish you well.

Many blessings,

FRANCIS WELLER

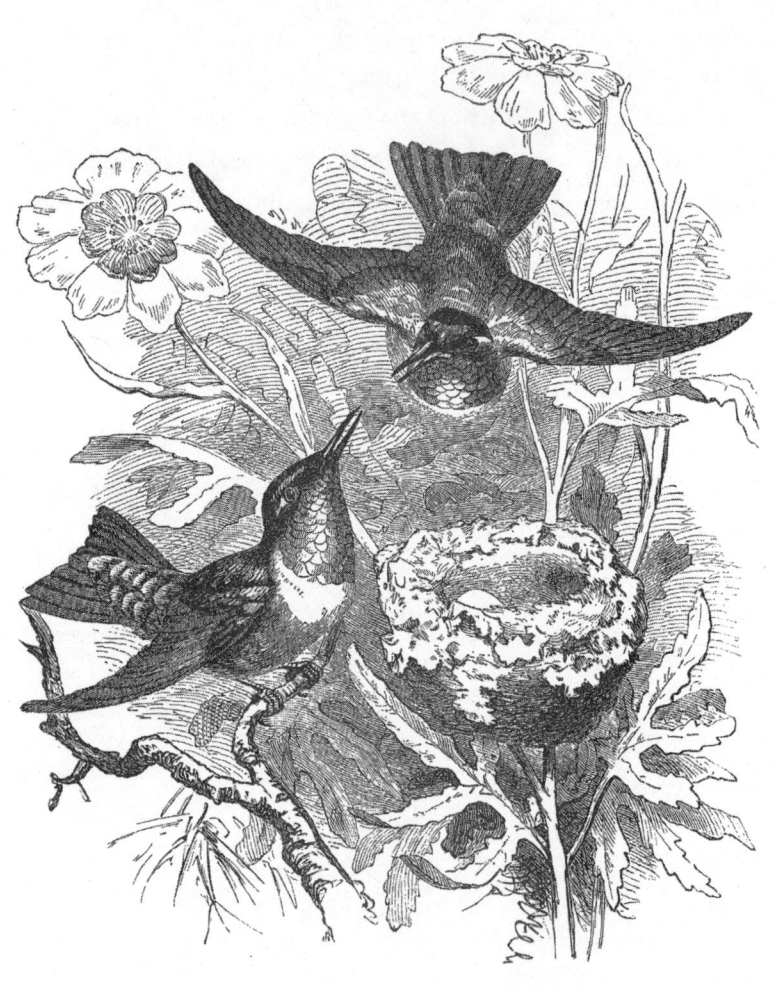

Seventeen

It All Turns on Affection

IT IS RAINING TONIGHT. What a blessed gift amid another potential drought year here in California. The air is sweet, the creeks are running, and the world goes on undeterred. Everything is in bud. We too are being readied for some new ripening. Whatever lies ahead will be shaped by the strength of our convictions. As poet-farmer Wendell Berry said, "It all turns on affection."[59] I believe this is true.

By saying it all turns on affection, I am saying that affection, love, a tender and fierce intimacy with the living world and our own mysterious depths are the most essential elements for us to cultivate in these tenuous times. In the absence of the ordinary, we thankfully have our own hearts to return to again and again. And here, in the secret nest of the heart, we can nourish a robust love for this world.

When asked what action was most important in dealing with climate disruption, Thich Nhat Hanh said, "What we most need to do is to hear within us the sounds of the earth crying."[60] This simple act is not so simple. To hear within us the sounds of the earth crying, we must develop the relational ground between us and the earth. We must become open and available to her sorrows and losses. We must be willing to join the Clan of the Brokenhearted.

Information will not be enough. We know the levels of CO_2 in the atmosphere. We know the percentage of old-growth forest remaining, and the number of elephants left in Africa. This is vital data, but not necessarily sufficient to warm the heart to feel the gravity of these facts.

Nor will moralism save the day. We won't necessarily feel moved to hear the cries of the earth because we *should*. We won't lean into the great work of cultural and ecosystem change because we *should*. We need the heart aroused, registering its fealty to our lives and the wider animate world. *We will protect what we love.* And so much needs our protection. Our affection needs to carry a potency capable of resisting careless and harmful actions directed at vulnerable communities and fragile ecosystems. Affection is not passive or necessarily gentle. It also carries a ferocity that enables us to stand up and protest, to advocate on behalf of what has been marginalized. As bell hooks said, "The practice of love is the most powerful antidote to the practice of domination."[61] She reminds us that love is a verb, and not only a feeling.

Loving the world is an act of courage. To lean into all that is circulating around the planet is to become porous to the rising tide of grief and sorrow, fear and trauma. This is the wedge through which we are broken open to our greater love for this beautiful, beleaguered world. Our intimacy with the world is felt within the folds of our vulnerability. Loving anyone or anything is a fierce and demanding practice. The Austrian poet Rainer Maria Rilke said that to love another "is perhaps the most diffi-cult of all our tasks, the ultimate, the last test and proof, the work for which all other work is but preparation."[62] Can we imagine that allowing our love to fall outward into the waiting arms of the world is what we have been preparing for? What if our love was meant to bless and nourish not only our immediate kin but also the wider expanse of otherness, the hills and creeks, prairie dogs and sparrows. Loving the world is no small thing.

When the heart unfurls through any kind of initiatory experience, we come to recognize that our identity is fused with all things. We are wed to the land around us, the migratory pathways, the hibernating creatures, the dormant seeds waiting for rain to fall and the sun to warm the soil. We are kin with EVERYTHING. Everything exists entangled with everything else.

In the absence of the ordinary, it falls to us to kindle bonds of kinship with all that is near to us. We are at a threshold for our world. In the days to come, everything we do will be significant. Never doubt that each of us is essential to the welfare of the commons. Everyone is a vector. Choose what you spread. It all turns on affection.

NOTES

1 Susan Murphy, *A Fire Runs Through All Things* (Boulder, CO: Shambhala, 2023), 41.

2 James Hillman, *Re-Visioning Psychology* (New York: Harper and Row, 1975), 16.

3 Martín Prechtel, *Long Life, Honey in the Heart* (New York: Tarcher/Putnam, 1999), 359.

4 Edward Tick, "Healing the Wounds of War," *Parabola*, October 31, 2014, *https://parabola.org/2014/10/31/healing-the-wounds-of-war/*.

5 Rebecca E. Phillips, "Ceremonial PTSD Therapies Favored by Native American Veterans," *WSU Insider*, June 17, 2014, *https://news.wsu.edu/2014/06/17/ceremonial-ptsd-therapies-favored-by-native-american-veterans/*.

6 Rainer Maria Rilke, quoted in Norman Brown, *Life Against Death: The Psychoanalytic Meaning of History* (Middletown, CT: Wesleyan University Press, 1959), 66.

7 Rainer Maria Rilke, *Rilke's Book of Hours: Love Poems to God*, trans. Anita Barrows and Joanna Macy (New York: Riverhead Books, 1996), 88.

8 Ira Progoff shared during a Journal Writing Intensive, Berkeley, California, 1981.

9 Jalaluddin Rumi, *Rumi: The Book of Love*, trans. Coleman Barks (New York: HarperCollins, 2003), 123.

10 Gautama Buddha, quoted in Mark Epstein, *The Trauma of Everyday Life* (New York: Penguin Books, 2013), 35.

11 Rumi, *Rumi: The Book of Love*, 137.

12 Jaime Gil de Biedma, Spanish poet, 1929–1990, Quotes, Goodreads, *www.goodreads.com/quotes/605378-i-believed-that-i-wanted-to-be-a-poet-but*.

13 For more information, see "Freedom and Choice" in Francis
    Weller, *The Wild Edge of Sorrow: Rituals of Renewal and the Sacred
    Work of Grief* (Berkeley, CA: North Atlantic Books, 2015), 157.

14 Rainer Maria Rilke, *Selected Poems of Rainer Maria Rilke*, trans.
    Robert Bly (New York: Harper and Row, 1981), 21.

15 Dante Alighieri, quoted in *The Heart Aroused: Poetry and the Pres-
    ervation of the Soul in Corporate America*, trans. David Whyte (New
    York: Doubleday, 1994), 1.

16 Jennifer Welwood, "The Dakini Speaks," JenniferWelwood.com,
    https://jenniferwelwood.com/poetry/the-dakini-speaks/.

17 Stanton Marlan, *The Black Sun: The Alchemy and Art of Darkness*
    (Dallas: Texas A&M University Press, 2003), 190.

18 Federico García Lorca, *In Search of the Duende*, trans. Christopher
    Maurer (New York: New Directions Books, 1998), 67.

19 Lorca, *In Search of the Duende*, 62.

20 Joan Halifax, *The Fruitful Darkness: Reconnecting with the Body of
    the Earth* (New York: HarperCollins, 1993), 5.

21 John O'Donohue, *Beauty: The Invisible Embrace* (New York:
    HarperCollins, 2004), 23.

22 O'Donohue, *Beauty*, 24.

23 Rilke, *Selected Poems of Rainer Maria Rilke*, 207.

24 Albertus Magnus, quoted in James Hillman, *Alchemical Psychology:
    Uniform Edition of the Writings of James Hillman* (Putnam, CT:
    Spring Publications, 2010), 38.

25 James Hillman, *Insearch: Psychology and Religion* (Putnam, CT:
    Spring Publications, 1967), 56.

26 Philalethes, quoted in James Hillman, *Alchemical Psychology:
    Uniform Edition of the Writings of James Hillman* (Putnam, CT:
    Spring Publications, 2010), 39.

27 C. G. Jung, quoted in James Hillman, *The Myth of Analysis: Three
    Essays in Archetypal Psychology* (New York: Harper Torchbooks,
    1972), 11.

28 C. G. Jung, *Psychology and Alchemy: Collected Works of C. G. Jung*,
    vol. 12 (Princeton, NJ: Princeton University Press, 1968), 167.

29 James Hillman, *Alchemical Psychology: Uniform Edition of the Writ-
    ings of James Hillman* (Putnam, CT: Spring Publications, 2010), 40.

30 Susan Mehrtens, "The Hardest of All Things," Jungian Center for the Spiritual Sciences, October 12, 2023, *https://jungiancenter.org/the -hardest-of-all-things/#_ftn6*.

31 Primary satisfactions are the undeniable and irrefutable needs of the psyche that were established over the long journey of our species and are imprinted in our beings as expectations awaiting fulfillment.

32 Gary Snyder, interviewed by Jonathan White, *Talking on the Water: Conversations about Nature and Creativity* (San Francisco: Sierra Club Books, 1994), 148.

33 Hillman, *Alchemical Psychology*, 63.

34 Elizabeth Marshall Thomas, *The Old Ways: A Story of the First People* (New York: Sarah Crichton Books, 2006), 10.

35 Robert Macfarlane, "Landspeak," *Orion*, May/June 2015, *https:// orionmagazine.org/article/landspeak/*.

36 James Cowan, *Letters from a Wild State: Rediscovering Our True Relationship to Nature* (New York: Bell Tower, 1991), 97.

37 Gautama Buddha, quoted in Sharon Salzberg, *Lovingkindness: The Revolutionary Art of Happiness* (Boston: Shambhala, 2020), 22.

38 Rumi, *Rumi: The Book of Love*, 179.

39 Rebecca del Rio's beautiful poem is used with the author's permission. "Prescription for the Disillusioned," Rebecca del Rio Poetry, *www.rebeccadelriopoetry.com/prescription-for-the-disillusioned*.

40 Paul Shepard, interviewed by Jonathan White, *Talking on the Water: Conversations about Nature and Creativity* (San Francisco: Sierra Club Books, 1994), 214.

41 R. D. Laing, *The Politics of Experience* (New York: Ballantine Books, 1971), 58.

42 Chellis Glendinning, *My Name Is Chellis and I'm in Recovery from Western Civilization* (Boston: Shambhala, 1994), 17.

43 Glendinning, *My Name Is Chellis*, 57.

44 David Hinton, *Hunger Mountain: A Field Guide to Mind and Land-scape* (Boston: Shambhala, 2012), 30.

45 Sigmund Freud, quoted in Theodore Roszak, *The Voice of the Earth: An Exploration of Ecopsychology* (New York: Simon and Schuster, 1992), 45.

46 Martin Shaw, shared at a lecture in Sebastopol, California, 2019.

47 Hinton, *Hunger Mountain*, 115.

48 Cowan, *Letters from a Wild State*, 8.

49 William Blake, *The Marriage of Heaven and Hell*, quoted in *News of the Universe: Poems of Twofold Consciousness*, chosen and introduced by Robert Bly (San Francisco: Sierra Club Books, 1980), 40.

50 Jay Griffiths, *Wild: An Elemental Journey* (New York: Jeremy P. Tarcher/Penguin, 2006), 22.

51 Griffiths, *Wild*, 25.

52 Brother David Steindl-Rast from a talk given in Marin County, California, 1995.

53 Kathleen Dean Moore, *Great Tide Rising* (Berkeley, CA: Counterpoint, 2016), 140.

54 C. G. Jung, quoted in Dolores LaChapelle, *Sacred Land, Sacred Sex, Rapture of the Deep: Concerning Deep Ecology and Celebrating Life* (Durango, CO: Kivaki Press, 1988), 73.

55 Deborah Eden Tull, *Luminous Darkness: An Engaged Buddhist Approach to Embracing the Unknown* (Boulder, CO: Shambhala, 2022).

56 David Whyte, Many Rivers Press newsletter, 2014.

57 Halifax, *Fruitful Darkness*.

58 C. G. Jung and Károly Kerényi, *Essays on a Science of Mythology* (London: Routledge & Kegan Paul, 1969), 92.

59 Wendell Berry, *It All Turns on Affection* (Berkeley, CA: Counterpoint, 2012).

60 Thich Nhat Hanh, quoted in *Spiritual Ecology: The Cry of the Earth*, ed. Llewellyn Vaughan-Lee (Point Reyes, CA: Golden Sufi Center, 2013), 245.

61 bell hooks, *Outlaw Culture: Resisting Representations* (London: Routledge, 2012), 281.

62 Rainer Maria Rilke, *Letters to a Young Poet* (New York: Penguin Books, 2013), 42.

BIBLIOGRAPHY

Berry, Wendell. *It All Turns on Affection*. Berkeley, CA: Counterpoint, 2012.

Blake, William. *The Marriage of Heaven and Hell*, quoted in *News of the Universe: Poems of Twofold Consciousness*. Chosen and introduced by Robert Bly. San Francisco: Sierra Club Books, 1980.

Brown, Norman. *Life Against Death: The Psychoanalytic Meaning of History*. Middletown, CT: Wesleyan University Press, 1959.

Cowan, James. *Letters from a Wild State: Rediscovering Our True Relationship to Nature*. New York: Bell Tower, 1991.

de Biedma, Jaime Gil. Quotes, Goodreads. *www.goodreads.com/quotes /605378-i-believed-that-i-wanted-to-be-a-poet-but*.

del Rio, Rebecca. "Prescription for the Disillusioned." Rebecca del Rio Poetry. *www.rebeccadelriopoetry.com/prescription-for-the -disillusioned*.

Epstein, Mark. *The Trauma of Everyday Life*. New York: Penguin Books, 2013.

Glendinning, Chellis. *My Name Is Chellis and I'm in Recovery from Western Civilization*. Boston: Shambhala, 1994.

Griffiths, Jay. *Wild: An Elemental Journey*. New York: Jeremy P. Tarcher/Penguin, 2006.

Halifax, Joan. *The Fruitful Darkness: Reconnecting with the Body of the Earth*. New York: HarperCollins, 1993.

Hillman, James. *Alchemical Psychology: Uniform Edition of the Writings of James Hillman*. Putnam, CT: Spring Publications, 2010.

Hillman, James. *The Myth of Analysis: Three Essays in Archetypal Psychology*. New York: Harper Torchbooks, 1972.

Hillman, James. *Insearch: Psychology and Religion*. Putnam, CT: Spring Publications, 1967.

Hillman, James. *Re-Visioning Psychology*. New York: Harper and Row, 1975.

Hinton, David. *Hunger Mountain: A Field Guide to Mind and Landscape*. Boston: Shambhala, 2012.

Hogan, Linda. *Dwellings: A Spiritual History of the Living World*. New York: Touchstone, 1995.

hooks, bell. *Outlaw Culture: Resisting Representations*. London: Routledge, 2012.

Jung, C. G. *Psychology and Alchemy: Collected Works of C. G. Jung*. Vol. 12. Princeton, NJ: Princeton University Press, 1968.

Jung, C. G., and Károly Kerényi. *Essays on a Science of Mythology*. London: Routledge & Kegan Paul, 1969.

LaChapelle, Dolores. *Sacred Land, Sacred Sex, Rapture of the Deep: Concerning Deep Ecology and Celebrating Life*. Durango, CO: Kivaki Press, 1988.

Laing, R. D. *The Politics of Experience*. New York: Ballantine Books, 1971.

Lorca, Federico García. *In Search of the Duende*. Translated by Christopher Maurer. New York: New Directions Books, 1998.

Macfarlane, Robert. "Landspeak." *Orion*, May/June 2015, *https:// orionmagazine.org/article/landspeak/*.

Marlan, Stanton. *The Black Sun: The Alchemy and Art of Darkness*. Dallas: Texas A&M University Press, 2003.

Mehrtens, Susan. "The Hardest of All Things." Jungian Center for the Spiritual Sciences, October 12, 2023. *https://jungiancenter.org /the-hardest-of-all-things/#_ftn6*.

Moore, Kathleen Dean. *Great Tide Rising*. Berkeley, CA: Counterpoint, 2016.

Murphy, Susan. *A Fire Runs Through All Things*. Boulder, CO: Shambhala, 2023.

O'Donohue, John. *Beauty: The Invisible Embrace*. New York: HarperCollins, 2004.

Phillips, Rebecca E. "Ceremonial PTSD Therapies Favored by Native American Veterans." *WSU Insider*, June 17, 2014, *https://news.wsu.edu/2014/06/17/ceremonial-ptsd-therapies-favored-by-native-american-veterans/*.

Prechtel, Martín. *Long Life, Honey in the Heart*. New York: Tarcher/Putnam, 1999.

Rilke, Rainer Maria. *Letters to a Young Poet*. New York: Penguin Books, 2013.

Rilke, Rainer Maria. *Rilke's Book of Hours: Love Poems to God*. Translated by Anita Barrows and Joanna Macy. New York: Riverhead Books, 1996.

Rilke, Rainer Maria. *Selected Poems of Rainer Maria Rilke*. Translated by Robert Bly. New York: Harper and Row, 1981.

Roszak, Theodore. *The Voice of the Earth: An Exploration of Ecopsychology*. New York: Simon and Schuster, 1992.

Rumi, Jalaluddin. *Rumi: The Book of Love*. Translated by Coleman Barks. New York: HarperCollins, 2003.

Salzberg, Sharon. *Lovingkindness: The Revolutionary Art of Happiness*. Boston: Shambhala, 2020.

Thomas, Elizabeth Marshall. *The Old Ways: A Story of the First People*. New York: Sarah Crichton Books, 2006.

Tick, Edward. "Healing the Wounds of War." *Parabola*, October 31, 2014. *https://parabola.org/2014/10/31/healing-the-wounds-of-war/*.

Tull, Deborah Eden. *Luminous Darkness: An Engaged Buddhist Approach to Embracing the Unknown*. Boulder, CO: Shambhala, 2022.

Vaughan-Lee, Llewellyn, ed. *Spiritual Ecology: The Cry of the Earth*. Point Reyes, CA: Golden Sufi Center, 2013.

Weller, Francis. *The Wild Edge of Sorrow: Rituals of Renewal and the Sacred Work of Grief*. Berkeley, CA: North Atlantic Books, 2015.

Welwood, Jennifer. "The Dakini Speaks." *JenniferWelwood.com*. *https://jenniferwelwood.com/poetry/the-dakini-speaks/*.

White, Jonathan White. *Talking on the Water: Conversations About Nature and Creativity*. San Francisco: Sierra Club Books, 1994.)

White, David. *The Heart Aroused: Poetry and the Preservation of the Soul in Corporate America*. New York: Doubleday, 1994.

Whyte, David. Many Rivers Press newsletter, 2014.

INDEX

ABOUT THE AUTHOR

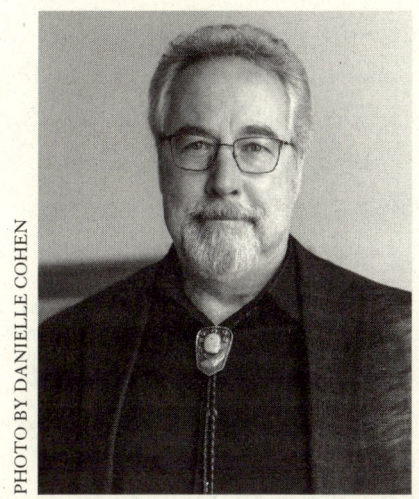

FRANCIS WELLER, MFT, is a psychotherapist, writer, and soul activist. He is a master of synthesizing diverse streams of thought from psychology, anthropology, mythology, alchemy, Indigenous cultures, and poetic traditions. Author of *The Wild Edge of Sorrow: Rituals of Renewal and the Sacred Work of Grief* and *The Threshold Between Loss and Revelation* (with Rashani Réa), he has introduced the healing work of ritual to thousands of people. He founded and directs WisdomBridge, an organization that offers educational programs that seek to integrate the wisdom from Indigenous cultures with the insights and knowledge gathered from Western poetic, psychological, and spiritual traditions.

For more than forty years, Francis has worked as a psychother-apist and developed a style he calls *soul-centered psychotherapy*. As a gifted therapist and teacher, he has been described as a jazz artist, improvising and moving fluidly in and out of deep emotional ter-ritories with groups and individuals, bringing imagination and attention to places often held with judgment and shame. His latest offerings are a ten-session audio series on *Living a Soulful Life and Why It Matters*, a four-session series on *An Apprenticeship with Sorrow: Community, Ritual, and the Sacred Work of Grief*, and a five-session series on *The Alchemy of Initiation: Soul Work and the Art of Ripening*.

Francis received a bachelor's degree from the University of Wisconsin–Green Bay and two master's degrees from John F. Kennedy University in clinical psychology and transpersonal psy-chology. His writings have appeared in anthologies and journals exploring the confluence between psyche, nature, and culture. His work was featured in *The Sun* magazine (October 2015), the *Utne Reader* (Fall 2016), and the *Kosmos Journal*. Francis is currently on staff at Commonweal Cancer Help Program, co-leading their weeklong retreats with Michael Lerner. He is completing his fourth book, *Facing the World with Soul and Why It Matters*.

For more information on upcoming workshops, to sign up for the newsletter, or to purchase books and audio series, please go to *www.francisweller.net*.

ABOUT
NORTH ATLANTIC BOOKS

North Atlantic Books (NAB) is an independent, nonprofit publisher committed to a bold exploration of the relationships between mind, body, spirit, and nature. Founded in 1974, NAB aims to nurture a holistic view of the arts, sciences, humanities, and healing. To make a donation or to learn more about our books, authors, events, and newsletter, please visit *www.northatlanticbooks.com*.